LETTERS TO A YOUNG DOCTOR

Praise for *Letters to a Young Doctor*

'A brilliant and impassioned cry from the heart at the current state of medical education and practice, from the top of the profession. That it is also spiritual, wise and funny makes this book something special.'

Jesse Norman MP, Financial Secretary to the Treasury, author of *The Big Society*

'A delightful and witty account of the life of a successful surgeon, whose own warmth and empathy has clearly defined his medical practice. His plea to revisit reforms in our health service – which rely on command and control and which are destroying the values of care and compassion – is timely and powerful. *Letters to a Young Doctor* is both a lively guide to young doctors and also a serious message to our society about the ways in which we are seeing the de-professionalising of great professions in pursuit of distorted notions of efficiency.'

Baroness Helena Kennedy QC

'At a time when, more than ever, we are focused on the NHS, this is a reminder of the compassionate care that needs to be at its heart. Part polemic, part guide to a medical career, and part memoir, *Letters to a Young Doctor* is also very funny and written with passion, elan and fluency. Dr Hilali Noordeen has written a book which should be prescribed reading for any budding doctor, not to mention their parents.'

Rachel Kelly, writer, mental health advocate and author of *Sunday Times* bestseller *Black Rainbow: How Words Can Heal: My Journey Through Depression*

LETTERS TO A YOUNG DOCTOR

Exploring and Surviving a Career in Medicine

DR HILALI NOORDEEN

First published in 2021 by whitefox

Copyright © Hilali Noordeen

The moral right of Hilali Noordeen to be identified as the author of this work has been asserted in accordance with the Copyright, Designs and Patents Act 1988.

All rights reserved. No part of this publication may be reproduced or transmitted in any form or by any means, electronic or mechanical including photocopying, recording or any information storage or retrieval system, without prior permission in writing from the publishers.

ISBN 978-1-913532-22-2

Also available as an ebook
ISBN 978-1-913532-23-9

Typeset by Seagulls design
Cover design by kid-ethic
Project management by whitefox
Printed and bound by CPI

For Suleyman, Ruqayyah and Haroun

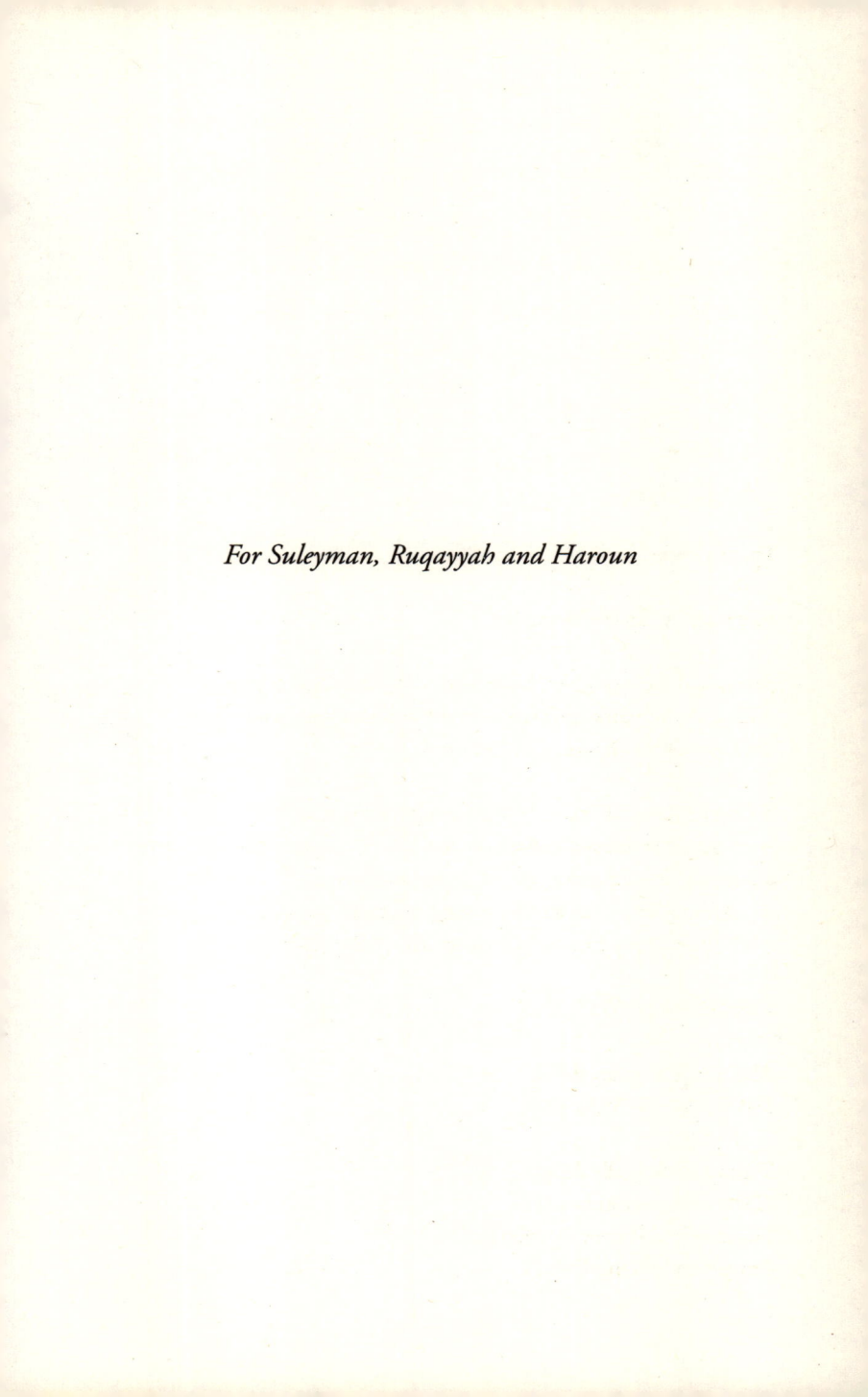

Contents

Foreword   xi

Part I – FIRST STEPS

Chapter One	Serendipity	2
Chapter Two	The Beginning (Education)	13
Chapter Three	The Middle (Training)	24
Chapter Four	The End (Practice)	37
Chapter Five	An Epidemic of Harm	54
Chapter Six	Opioids Have Become the Religion of the Masses	64
Chapter Seven	The Crowning Virus That Changed Everything	75

Part II – THE CRISIS

Chapter Eight	Alienation	82
Chapter Nine	Culture of Care or Command and Control?	91
Chapter Ten	The Big Society: Re-establishing Care over Control	102
Chapter Eleven	Groundhog Day	111
Chapter Twelve	Introspection – A Return to the Spirit	115

Bibliography   142

Foreword

'Dad, I think I want to study medicine, just like you. What do you think?'

Taken aback by my fifteen-year-old son's unexpected announcement, I knew I must think carefully about my answer. I explained that I needed time and would respond in due course. But why was I taken aback? That was what I had to ask myself, before issuing any form of response. It gradually dawned on me that I was worried my son had all the best intentions, and was going into medicine for all the right reasons, but the profession of modern medicine was no longer true to itself. Somehow, the practice of medicinal care had lost its way. Modern doctors practised their profession as if it were only a science and no longer an art: using their minds, their instruments, their medicines, their algorithms and processes, but not their hearts. Did I really want my son to enter into a profession that was almost bound to disillusion him, and betray his noble aspirations?

I meditated upon this conundrum. I, like many others, embarked on a career in medicine because I cared deeply for humanity, which I saw as part of my extended family. I earnestly wished to alleviate suffering. I was fired by a perhaps utopian idealism, hoping that I could, even if in a tiny way, enhance the health and well-being of my fellow human beings, and remove physical suffering while simultaneously showing compassion and care to my patients, alleviating their anxieties and lifting their sense of vulnerability. I am certain that the vast majority of students who undertake medicine do so with the expectation of delivering care with compassion and genuine concern. What is also true is that the vast majority of students go into medicine knowing very little about what the current practice of medicine entails. Some, of course, are the children of physicians like myself, but even they have only a fleeting idea of the reality of medical practice, and certainly would know little about the practice of disciplines outside those of their parents or their parents' friends.

Having meditated on my son's question, I thought that, rather than offer him platitudes and possibly conflicting advice, I would write him a manual. It was to be at once a meditation and description of the current practice of modern medicine and a document identifying the inherent problems, while suggesting solutions that might help him make a difference. In the Eastern tradition, simple parables are often used to illustrate fundamental truths. As the child becomes an adult, the same story reveals more complex messages. This is different from the modern Western tradition where, as children grow older, they are told different stories with greater complexity.

In the course of writing the book, I became increasingly reliant on the advice of my dear friend Reza Shah-Kazemi, Research Associate at the Institute of Ismaili Studies in London, and an authority and author on the Universalist perspective of spirituality. His contribution has been essential to this book.

I sent a preliminary draft of my manual to a close friend, whose daughter I knew also wanted to apply for a career in medicine. My friend, Rachel Kelly (a published author herself), told me that what I had to say would attract not only an audience of innumerable students wishing to study medicine, but also their parents, who might wish to know what their children were letting themselves in for. I enlisted the help of the brilliant Bryony Sutherland, who, in a preliminary analysis of my first chapter, got me thinking further about what I was really attempting to say and how I should say it. The challenge was to say it in a way that would make sense to an adolescent and to an adult. I have treated children all my working life, and have always addressed them, rather than their parents, for two reasons. First, pragmatically, I needed them to 'buy in' to their treatment. Second, if the children understood what was being said, then their parents would too.

While I was preparing the book for presentation, with my wonderful agent Elizabeth Sheinkman, along came the novel coronavirus SARS-CoV-2 – the crowning virus, which has changed the way in which all doctors work, and is likely to have a profound effect on the way in which we deliver care, and the way we live, for the foreseeable future. She asked me to write about it and I did, for the problems that we face with coronavirus apply across all medicine

I was convinced that the answers lay in the heart, in the human spirit – that spirit that makes us all as one in the deepest root of our humanity. I firmly believe all traditions are united on certain essential principles and values, and differ only in their modes of application. I am therefore a 'perennialist' at heart, who believes in the immensely positive role that has been performed throughout history by the spiritual underpinnings of these great traditions. More importantly, I believe that it is only through embracing this spiritual patrimony that we can address and solve the interrelated crises afflicting the contemporary world.

This book, therefore, is for my sons and my daughter, who may also wish to enter into the study of medicine. It is also for all the sons and daughters and all the aspiring students who are considering embarking on the study of medicine and also for those already enmeshed in their respective medical careers, hopefully to give them a guide for an ever-changing landscape, providing not only a critique of modern medicine but also some pointers towards possible solutions to the crisis, both practical and spiritual. The book is therefore divided into two distinct parts. **FIRST STEPS**, aimed more at the aspirant, identifies the tools required for longevity in the profession, and functions as a working 'manual' of sorts, to be used throughout their career. The second part, **CRISIS**, addresses the issues facing the young practising doctor, which the aspirant may only come across once well *into* their career, empowering them with the resources to survive the inevitable questions that will arise and may periodically challenge their prospect of survival within their chosen path.

I wish all future medical practitioners all the very best on this journey, with all of its twists and turns.

Part I

FIRST STEPS

CHAPTER ONE

Serendipity

There is a tide in the affairs of men,
Which, taken at the flood, leads on to fortune;
Omitted, all the voyage of their life
Is bound in shallows and in miseries.
On such a full sea are we now afloat,
And we must take the current when it serves,
Or lose our ventures.
***Julius Caesar* by Shakespeare**

The Oxford English Dictionary defines serendipity as 'The occurrence and development of events by chance in a happy and beneficial way'. We underestimate the role of serendipity in our lives, and instead attribute success to our own genius. Each one of us has innate but different abilities, and there is no doubt that to benefit from an opportunity requires effort.

It is one thing to make an effort to 'take it at the flood'; it is another to recognise the nature of the tide. However, it is an altogether different matter to give credence to tides at all. It is akin to being unaware of, or at least ignoring, the effect of the phases of the moon on tides.

The first use of the word 'serendipity' in the English language was by Horace Walpole in 1754, in a letter he wrote to his friend Horace Mann, where he explained the unexpected discovery he had made by reference to a Persian fairy tale, *The Three Princes of Serendip*. These princes were 'always making discoveries, by accidents and sagacity, of things that they were not in quest of'. The name comes from Serendip, used by Arab traders as an old name for my native Sri Lanka. Its derivation is from the Sanskrit and has been exported into many languages, broadly meaning 'fortunate chance'.

Serendipity in science cannot be underestimated. It plays an integral role in research and discoveries at all times. Most discoveries are there to be made, but can only be made by minds that are prepared to receive them. As Louis Pasteur famously stated, 'Chance favours the prepared mind'. Most scientific discoveries are made accidentally during the course of investigations, and are often unexpected, the products of induction. An excellent example of a serendipitous observation, which led to a discovery of unfathomable proportions, is that of Alexander Fleming in 1928. He was suffering from a bad cold and unexpectedly sneezed into a Petri dish full of bacteria, which he left on his desk without intent. When he came back some days later, he noticed to his surprise that the bacteria in the dish had been completely destroyed. His curiosity was aroused and, following his instinct, he worked to isolate, for the first time, the antibacterial protein found in tears and mucus. Convinced that more important agents existed, he began searching for other environmental antibacterials, eventually coming up with penicillin in 1928, for which he won the Nobel Prize. Fleming commented: 'Nature makes penicillin, I just found it; one sometimes finds what one is not looking for.'

There are many examples like this, all of which go to prove that scientific discovery is not always, as is often assumed, a process of thesis and antithesis, or thesis and experimentation leading to a synthesis of information, or thesis based on inductive logic that is then tested by means of experimentation to either refute or confirm the hypothesis. It is usually a simple case of a serendipitous observation that subsequently leads to a thesis, which is then tested.

Such is the case with a career, or indeed a life. Our choices are often influenced by a chance meeting, encounter, or conversation. In modern days, it may even be as a consequence of a chance internet trawl. We may not credit it as such, but it is often a serendipitous decision.

So it was in the case of my career. While I was at school studying for my A levels, I couldn't think of anything that I would really like to do. I ended up settling on a degree in chemistry, because this was the subject that interested me most, having studied maths, physics and chemistry for my A levels. However, when I got to Oxford University, it soon became obvious to me, having attended the first term of lectures and tutorials, that chemistry at A level was one thing, but chemistry at degree level, a subject of academic study, was an entirely different matter. This bothered me a great deal and I decided to change my course to that of physiological sciences, which held much more interest for me.

By chance, I met a fellow student at my college (which only had three or four medical students a year), who happened to live on my staircase. We became friends and enjoyed many conversations together. In the course of our discussions, he related to me that he came from a family of doctors, and it seemed to him natural that he should also continue in this tradition. I, on the other hand, came from a family of businessmen, not one of whom was a professional of any sort. In fact, I was the first in my family to go to university at all. We talked at length and I became increasingly fascinated with medicine, but then was surprised to learn that he no longer wished to practise it! He was much more interested in the humanities and told me confidentially that he intended to leave medicine and change courses. He was worried as to whether the college would let him do so, because that would mean an enormous loss of income both for the college and for the university, as being a medical student was, and remains, a massive source of funding. Since Oxford had only one hundred medical students, each one of them had tremendous economic value. I immediately volunteered to take his place on the GMC Register, thus saving the college money and resources.

My friend and I went to see the Dean together and made this offer to him, which initially took him aback, but then he saw the sense of it and discussed the matter with the university. He announced this was indeed a possibility, except that I would have to sit a special paper to satisfy the university's minimum requirement of an A level pass in either zoology or biology to qualify as a medical student (I had neither). I undertook tutorials in zoology, and managed to pass my A level (just) within one term. Thus, I became a medical student and my friend became a student of the humanities (I think he went on to read politics, philosophy and economics).

We met several years afterwards at a gaudy, or reunion, and fell on each other with great hugs and affection, thanking each other profusely for the opportunity. He had by that time become the CEO of a telecoms firm. And so my own career in medicine was serendipitous, as was his career in the telecoms industry. These serendipitous occurrences have continued throughout my career, and no doubt in many careers.

• • •

On many occasions after a good night out, I persuaded my more earnest fellow students to sign me in, which had an unfortunate consequence. My anatomy viva was undertaken by the Professor of Anatomy himself, in subfusc – suit, bow tie and gown. This was a spectacle indeed. The viva examinations were effectively the students demonstrating the human body to their tutors. This offered the strange sight of both the tutor, in his rather splendid gown, and the students, in their gowns, suits and bow ties (usually white), standing over bodies. It soon became abundantly clear to the Professor of Anatomy that he hadn't seen me very often in the anatomy demonstrations. To add insult to injury, in the process of demonstrating the function of the arm, I accidently smeared the arm and its formaldehyde over the professor's gown. The result was catastrophic in that he failed me in anatomy. I was thus forced to undertake a two-month course in human anatomy during the summer vacation. I had been invited to spend that summer travelling around the States with the most beautiful girl, and this imposition was a crushing blow.

However, all was not lost. Much to my initial horror, during my summer holiday I was banished to Leeds, and joined the large number of Scandinavian medical students gathering at the same institution over the summer. (I was told that the number of Scandinavian bodies donated to science, and therefore available for dissection, was few indeed.) My horror turned to joy as I discovered that the vast majority of Scandinavian students were female. On my table, upon which was a cadaver that we dissected from top to bottom, were four beautiful female medical students, one of whom was showing a particular interest in me. I recall that our hands met while dissecting the lesser omentum, and the rest of my stay in Leeds was most pleasant.

While I was a student, I undertook my orthopaedic training at the Nuffield Orthopaedic Centre in Oxford, under the formidable Robert Duthie, previously Professor of Orthopaedics in Pittsburgh for fifteen years, who had trained mainly with the great luminaries of orthopaedics in the United States. He was a dour Scotsman and there is an apocryphal story about him, where one trainee, on being shown a horrific injury, exclaimed 'My God!' Without hesitation, Professor Duthie replied, 'No, simply Professor Duthie.'

Duthie's medical students had not only to accompany his junior staff on ward rounds and Saturday teaching rounds but also, at the end of their four-week stint with him, take a formal graduate examination in orthopaedics. In all the fifteen years Duthie had been there, no medical student had ever failed. I passed the written exam with flying colours, but I hadn't been to many practical demonstrations – a consequence of my being President of the Oxford Union during that time – and this showed when it came to my practical examination. We were examined by an external examiner, Professor George Bentley from University College London, who was at the time one of the foremost educators. At the end of my examination, he commented to me that it was clear I hadn't examined many patients from an orthopaedic point of view. I concurred with him and he failed me. The first medical student ever to have failed under the aegis of Professor Duthie at Oxford.

I was summoned to see the Dean, and he told me that this was indeed bad form, and that Professor Duthie was upset and baying for me to repeat the whole year. He told me that the only way I could redeem myself was to be Professor Duthie's personal assistant during the forthcoming four-week Easter vacation and write an essay each week, after which Professor Bentley would be summoned to come and re-examine just me, to ensure that I was of sufficient standard to pass the exams. This happened. Professor Bentley informed me that I had passed extremely well. In the interim, I had written a mini-thesis that pleased Professor Duthie, and at the end of my stint with him, he asked me whether I had ever considered a career in orthopaedics, to which I replied in the affirmative. He sent me to Massachusetts General Hospital to do an elective in orthopaedics.

Many years later, once I had qualified and was up for my registrar interviews, I was interviewed at the Royal National Orthopaedic Hospital in Stanmore, and the Chairman of the Interview Committee was none other than Professor George Bentley. He asked me, as he did everyone else, how I came upon a career in orthopaedics. I told him, got the job and have remained there ever since as registrar, senior lecturer and now consultant. So, a serendipitous failure was a pillar of my success.

* * *

When I was a newly appointed spinal surgeon at the Royal National Orthopaedic Hospital, at the Children's Hospital in Great Ormond Street and at the Middlesex Hospital, I was invited by an instrument company in the US both to give a lecture on my work and to have a tour of their facilities. They booked me on a business-class British Airways flight (my first), and made arrangements for my accommodation, dinner and talk. It was a simple one-night stay and I arrived at Heathrow, cutting it fine as I often do. They checked me in without any difficulty as I was flying business class and had only hand luggage. As I was rushing towards the gate, I realised I did not have a tie, and I stopped at Harrods for ten minutes to buy one. I arrived at the gate approximately twenty-five minutes before the plane was due to take off. By this time they had closed the external doors but not the plane door. They told me they had offloaded me, as I only had hand luggage, and there was no possibility of getting 'back' on the plane.

This was the only flight to Memphis that day, and my arguments fell on deaf ears. I was devastated. I went a floor down to the ticketing office. They made sympathetic sounds and told me that the only way I could get to Memphis on time was to leave on a flight to JFK Airport in New York that was due to take off in an hour, and then take a connecting flight to Memphis from LaGuardia Airport. However, I would have no more than twenty minutes to get to LaGuardia. I said that I would try anything, so this is what they arranged for me.

I rushed over to the New York flight and boarded it without incident. I was sitting in business class, seething, and reading a book. An announcement came over the tannoy, asking whether there was anyone qualified to offer medical aid. My first instinct, as always in these circumstances, was to dive deeper into my book and not offer my services, usually from a feeling of modesty, on the grounds that I was sure there would be others on the plane who would be much better qualified to give the sort of assistance required. Given that I was a surgeon, I did not feel qualified to treat a heart attack or asthma attack, as I had last dealt with these common conditions years before, as a medical student. A few minutes passed, and then the captain of the plane approached me with the manifest in his hands.

'It says here that you are a doctor. Is this true?' I replied that I was, but that it was extremely unlikely that I would be able to help, since most of my work involved a sterile theatre, lights and instruments. I asked him to please search for someone who would be more qualified, but if he failed then of course he could ask me.

A few moments later, the captain returned. 'Well, we are at the point of having to land at Reykjavik Airport.'

This alarmed me greatly, as it would spell the end of my speech in Memphis. I immediately volunteered to help.

The captain explained that there was a lady on the plane who was thought to be pregnant and who had gone into urinary retention (the inability to pass urine), to the extent that her bladder was so full she was about to collapse. There was apparently a nurse on the plane, but she did not know how to pass in a urinary catheter. We were moved to an empty spot just behind the captain's cabin, and in that area they did in fact have a urinary catheter on board. Apparently, many drunken male passengers, particularly those with prostate issues, go into urinary retention while flying. Therefore, British Airways always carried a catheter. They also had some antiseptic on board. I cleaned the area, passed in the urinary catheter, and drained more than one litre of fluid. I blew up the balloon in the catheter, so that the catheter remained in place, and told the patient that she should get further investigations and treatment, because this was extremely unusual. I put her safely back into her seat, catheter in place, with strict instructions not to remove it until she got to a hospital, and went back to my seat with my book, greatly relieved that the flight had not been interrupted.

The captain returned, this time with a large duty-free selection in tow. He offered me whatever I wished. I told him the story of what had happened and why I needed to get to LaGuardia, and he told me that he would take me to the front of the plane as soon as we landed, but also let the JFK authorities know that I had this problem, and he was sure that they would help. I just urged him to try and get the plane as fast as possible into JFK so that I had as much time as possible to get to LaGuardia. He happily agreed. Nevertheless, he insisted that I take some duty-free, and he explained to me that I had in fact saved British Airways approximately £250,000. I asked him how so, and he said:

1. He would have had to dump approximately £50,000 worth of fuel.
2. He would have had to pay landing and take-off rights in Reykjavik, which amounted to another £50,000.

3. He would have had to refuel (another £50,000).
4. He estimated the cost of late tickets, hotels stays etc, being approximately another £100,000.

Pleased to have been of assistance, I helped myself to the duty-free, having rejected it up until that point. He then asked me whether there was anything else I would like, and I said that I had never travelled first class, and would love to have the experience. He put me into first class and also put an endorsement on my Executive Club Card that meant I was upgraded to first class for approximately a year thereafter, on any flight that I took. This was a most serendipitous pleasure.

We arrived at JFK. I was met at the front of the plane by the Airport Chief, who took me straight to the front of the queue at Immigration, announcing: 'This doctor has just saved a woman's life.' I was immediately given an entry stamp – those of you familiar with Immigration at JFK will understand that this was nothing short of a miracle – and then taken to a waiting car with flashing yellow lights, which cruised through the blisteringly heavy traffic between JFK and LaGuardia. I was early for my flight.

I received the most incredible email in June 2016, which went as follows, with sections deleted to protect its author's anonymity:

Dear Dr Noordeen,

Let me re-introduce myself, nineteen years after we first met aboard a British Airways flight from London to New York (9/22/1997). I was a very distraught passenger with urinary retention and you graciously agreed to catheterize me, with the disclaimer that you had not done that since medical school. At the time you also recommended a number of tests to rule out multiple sclerosis (please see attached document).

An MRI of the brain revealed the presence of white matter hyperintensity. Since you are an orthopaedic surgeon, let me add that I was also diagnosed with cervical arthritis, which remained asymptomatic for the next eight years, and then developed into bilateral neck pain and upper extremity pain. I then became a patient at the [...] Center for Spine Health, and I am currently a patient at [...] Spine Center. My most recent MRI reveals reversal of cervical lordosis and multi-level disc disease.

Back to the brain issue, which is the reason why I write to you today. Following your suggestions, I did a spinal tap which excluded MS, a diagnosis which was later confirmed at the [...] Center for Multiple Sclerosis. I mention this hospital in [...] repeatedly because I became a cancer patient there in 2004. The white matter hyperintensity issue was set aside (the neurologist who performed a spinal tap irresponsibly described those as 'beauty marks of the brain'), until a couple of months ago when a neurologist I saw at the [...] Center for Brain Health in Las Vegas attributed it to a vascular condition that could explain the mild cognitive decline that I have experienced. My mother is an end-stage Alzheimer's patient and I am very concerned about my own neurological future.

To conclude, I want to thank you for initiating a diagnostic process that led to the discovery of a medical condition that demands my constant vigilance. In other news, since we met, I completed a Doctorate at Yale and I am a Professor of Film Studies at [...].

Sincerely,

(.....)

Serendipity.

CHAPTER TWO

The Beginning (Education)

When I arrived at Oxford University, the mission of the vast majority of my contemporaries was to join the Civil Service. The Civil Service had also been the primary aim of most of my contemporaries in school. It was incredibly difficult to get into, but more than anything else, it was also totally meritocratic. It depended on your performance in the challenging Civil Service exams.

The Civil Service had for centuries been the means of social change. A student of modest means could gain state-supported entry into a good university and, having subsequently experienced a good education and submitted a good performance in the Civil Service exams, enter the Civil Service. He or she could rise up the ranks to become either an ambassador or a permanent secretary, heading the various departments, which could lead to a knighthood and possibly, in some cases, the House of Lords. Given his or her broad experience, he or she could then serve on many committees and provide sterling service to the country.

This was particularly important in a society that was class-driven. The Civil Service was a great leveller, but, more than that, it gave everyone the possibility of transcending the social class they were born into and moving, through their own merits, into the upper echelons of government, social status and the House of Lords. What a marvellous institution!

This all changed while I was at Oxford. With the enormous salaries that even a young trainee in the City of London commanded, I found that, gradually, most of my contemporaries who would have aspired to join the Civil Service instead went to the City – where, it was often relayed to me, money had to be the reward in a system that created money! – and to various jobs as traders, brokers or bankers to achieve the social mobility that money would give them. This was a tremendous tragedy.

It is becoming clear that this class of commercial trainee and practitioner was potentially the problem, as opposed to those who created wealth. The banks lent vast sums of money without any concern about whether or how this money could be paid back, and a new wave of debt was created. There was, of course, a great deal of corruption in the institutions, with insider trading and the fixing of interest rates, but, fundamentally, irresponsible lending caused the creation of a whole class of virtual trades.

As the City and monetary institutions shrank after the 2008 credit crunch, the traditional professions, including the Civil Service, law and medicine, became increasingly popular. It is therefore imperative to the new generation of aspirants that whoever enters a profession enters it knowing what it entails and makes a decision to go into said profession based on the reality, rather than a triumph of hope.

• • •

Medicine is as much an art as it is a science, governed by the method involving hypothesis, thesis, antithesis and synthesis. It is often forgotten that the beginning of all scientific method is intuitive and starts with a hypothesis that may have no evidence. It is simply a 'hunch'. Whether it be the discovery of penicillin or the Theory of Relativity, the means by which the authors put forward these hypotheses was by definition not empirical, in that it could not be measured.

Medicine is an art because it involves an appreciation of the human body – which is art itself – and the human condition. The cues by which this appreciation occurs cannot be measured. Medicine is thus, in its essence, a craft whose tenets are learnt by means of an apprenticeship. The apprenticeship continues until the apprentice himself becomes the master.

Today, medical teaching involves a pre-clinical stage, a study of the basic sciences, which usually takes two years, but may also involve a further year of more fundamental study of the subject, leading to either a Bachelor of Science degree or a Bachelor of Arts degree (usually at Oxford or Cambridge University). Many universities allow this third year to be used for study outside mainstream medicine – for example, law, history or another similar subject. Some universities now combine the teaching of the basic sciences with that of the clinical, or practical, teaching of skills. In the US, a pre-requirement for entry into medical school is a bachelor's degree that involves human biology, chemistry and physics to some extent. This is then followed by an intensive four years of a medical degree, of which approximately two years involve the teaching of the basic sciences of anatomy, physiology, biochemistry and pharmacology, followed by approximately two years of the teaching of clinical skills.

The basic two years are common to all courses of medicine and involve the study of anatomy, physiology, biochemistry and pharmacology. Fundamentally, this is anatomy and physiology: anatomy being the study of the structure of the human body, and physiology the understanding of its function. In any university, these are by far the most challenging years, as a great deal of information needs to be assimilated so the understanding of structure and function can be as comprehensive as possible. A tall order to achieve in a period of two years! Nevertheless, it did not stop the likes of me, who enjoyed the social life in Oxford to an enormous extent, which made the anatomy 'demonstrations' – dissection of the human body – challenging at 9 a.m., particularly since the dissections were usually undertaken on bodies pickled in pungent-smelling formalin. Difficult to digest, after an early breakfast following a late night!

I now believe it would be more sensible to hold these demonstrations at midday and perhaps use modern technology to simulate the body, rather than the poor pickled specimens. As so many bodies are donated to science, I hope by now better methods exist for their preservation and disposal thereafter.

* * *

A darkness has descended into medical education. Education as a means has become an end.

The reign of quantity occurs at school under the guise of scientific method. Anything that is 'real' is something that is measurable. There is a misunderstanding that scientific method is the same as an experiment. In an experiment, by its very definition, it is important to be able to measure all the variables. The experiment is the means. It is not scientific method. Scientific method begins with intuition and ends with experiment. This distinction is little understood and, as a result, this reign of quantity pervades the very core of medicine. A triumph of means, that of measurement, over end; that of confirmation or refutation of an idea or a hypothesis. Yet, in reality, medicine is an art, as it requires an understanding of expression, of emotion and of empathy.

During any form of scientific teaching, any understanding of the issue of the philosophy of science – which is based in art or in the art of reason, imagination, intuition and memory – is ignored at best and decried at worst. Imagination, intuition and memory are consigned to being mere shadows of reality as opposed to the reality itself. We are governed by phenomena and the whole focus of our teaching method is similarly focused on the measurement of phenomena.

However, I am deeply grateful to my university and to my college at Oxford University for my education. The mainstay of my education consisted of one-to-one tutorials. I was taught first not to just look in a textbook, but to understand what my tutors were trying to teach me. This required a careful appreciation of every single word that was uttered during the course of a tutorial. I was taught to deconstruct each topic or issue to its basic form and to reconstruct it in ways I could understand. The whole of medicine was taught by an understanding of the fundamentals of medical science, almost an understanding of the philosophy of science and the philosophy of scientific method. I must admit I was a poor student and perhaps I did not spend long enough listening to the pearls of wisdom that were cast my way. Nevertheless, what little pearls I received have been the mainstay of my life and medical practice, and have enabled me to deconstruct and reconstruct every exam I have ever taken with consummate ease.

What seemed effortless was in fact the seed of understanding that was implanted in me at the outset by my excellent tutors at Balliol College, Paddy Phizackerley, Denis Noble and Gillian Morriss-Kay. Denis Noble was a brilliant cardiac physiologist, who made me understand the fundamentals of all neural activity, and Gillian Morriss-Kay taught me embryology, which is part of anatomy and is the science of the formation of human tissue from its origin. She described this as the basis of all anatomy, and how right she was. The understanding of the human form, from the clot to a fully formed embryo, has led me to a profound understanding and appreciation of both the structure and the beauty of human anatomy.

When Paddy Phizackerley died, Denis Noble wrote the most beautiful memorial to him. It began with the vision of Julian of Norwich repeating her vision of Jesus: 'all manner of things shall be well'. This is one of the most explicit expositions of the Universalist perspective in Christianity. Paddy was just that. An outstanding tutor who was principally responsible for my academic progress, and a man with tremendous vision. One able to understand my strengths and weaknesses: bolster my strengths, and mitigate my weaknesses.

To all three tutors, I am ever grateful. Most of all, I am grateful to this system, which has been in existence for several centuries, and taught so many of us. It is interesting to reflect that there are only three or four medical students at Balliol College every year, and among their alumni are Nobel Prize winners and numerous presidents of the Royal Colleges of Medicine and of Surgery. They must be doing something right.

The ability to learn at that level of intensity and to communicate one-to-one at an early stage in one's career and development is not a luxury but a necessity. There starts the idea of an apprenticeship. The idea of master and pupil. The head of Balliol College was in fact called 'Master', and at the end of every term there was a handshake in which tutors literally shook our hands and personally discussed our progress during the course of each term. Again, this was on a one-to-one basis, and a tremendous privilege.

* * *

Following the first years of the basic sciences, there then follow approximately three more years of clinical medicine in the UK, or two years in the US, the end result of which is a bachelor's degree in medicine and in surgery in the UK, or a doctorate of medicine in the US. In England, a doctor of medicine is usually a higher degree based on research, or an honorary degree. The doctorate of medicine ranks among the highest degrees awarded by Oxford University, and doctors of medicine are in the forefront of the degree ceremony and invited in perpetuity to any and every degree ceremony. There is also a benefaction of my college that obliges the college to treat me to lunch, should I wish to attend any of these ceremonies!

During our clinical attachment at medical school, we were taught that 90 per cent of all diagnoses could be made by means of a history (70 per cent) and an examination (20 per cent) alone. Investigations added only approximately 10 per cent, simply to confirm the diagnosis or to refute it. The current fashion of using algorithms to make a diagnosis has removed the responsibility to interact with the patient and to truly take a history. Freud had a view that a patient betrays (or reveals?) himself 'through every pore':

He that has eyes to see and ears to hear may convince himself that no mortal can keep a secret. If his lips are silent, he chatters with his fingertips; betrayal oozes out of him through every pore.

The very 'pore' that communicated the science and art of medicine from master or tutor to pupil is the same communication that occurs between a patient and a doctor. Strangely, the patient becomes the master and the doctor the pupil. It is only in this way that the nature of a patient's ailment can be understood. To understand the ailment, and thus to diagnose it, is halfway towards finding a remedy.

The examination of a patient also requires a 'bedside manner'. This necessitates a degree of empathy, kindness and understanding to truly elicit physical signs that may be clues to a diagnosis. The blink of an eyelid, the expression on a face. Much is not said and yet facial expression reveals everything. A grimace, a wince, often subtle, and yet so poignant. This wonderful method has now been replaced by a checklist of evidence, boxes that, if left unticked, remain open to criticism: red flags.

The apprenticeship necessary to understand the human subject requires many years. I have never stopped learning. It is hardly surprising that, for time immemorial in England, and in fact in the British Isles, surgeons who were ever apprentices would jealously guard their title of 'Mr' and belong to a guild, the Guild of Barber Surgeons. This was not simply a prejudice but a deep conviction that the art of human interaction that may potentially cure by means of surgery could only be undertaken, in terms of both understanding and skill, by means of an apprenticeship. The Fellowship of the Royal College of Surgeons is precisely that. Upon receiving this certificate from our guild, we cease to be doctors and become a 'Mister' or 'Miss'. This remains the case to this day. Most of us, even academic surgeons, would fight much harder to retain the title of 'Mr' or 'Miss' rather than 'Professor'. It is a badge of honour.

It is quite possible for education to be undertaken via reading a book, sitting in front of a screen or by some form of Skype call. I am deeply grateful for my education, which was by one-to-one human interaction. This is not to say that one cannot learn collectively at lectures, but even a lecture is an interaction between an individual and his audience. It has a different dynamic, but nevertheless it is in the realms of human interaction. It is also a three-dimensional interaction. It is not only an insight into what is being portrayed on a screen but an intuitive understanding of what is really being said.

How shall we make education beautiful? Or rather: how shall beauty bring out the positive aspects of our modern education system, and expel the darkness that is invading it? The main method at our disposal is the written and the spoken word. Poetry becomes words in motion. It becomes beauty in motion. A dark Shakespearean play nevertheless expresses beauty, even in murder, through cadence and the delivery of words. So it is with education. It is not difficult for this to be expressed both by text and visually, particularly in this day and age. There is a complex intelligence and imagination in cell division and in differentiation to live as an organ cell with blood cells, all starting from a single cell. There is beauty in the mystery of this transition and the breathtaking ability of its evolution to form a myriad of infinite possibilities. The complexity that individual organs both develop and mature is therefore art unfolding, and yet an infinitude of cells, each a universe in itself, a universe of function and structure. There is beauty in a cell, be it red or white, or indeed in the double-helical structure of DNA. The external universe of the stars is measured in the universe of the DNA and the universe of the single cell. The universe of the single atom. The universe of an electron, a proton, and so on. An entire universe is encapsulated in a single cell. These magnificent structures can be visualised both macroscopically and microscopically. One can behold the beauty of an ultrasound scan of a foetus, repeated at each stage, as the foetus grows into a newborn.

Let us repeat: virgin nature opens us up to the spiritual archetypes of beauty. The human body, from the simplest cell to the complexity of the brain, evokes the quintessence not only of the human being, but of the secret of virgin nature, the secret of creation as it emerges, fresh-minted, from the Hands of the Creator – as yet untouched by the hands of man. We are given a glimpse into the mystery of the human being as the 'microcosm', the 'small world', as well as a teaching about the nature of ailments and their remedy, in the following lines of a poem by Imam Ali (cousin and son-in-law of the Prophet Muhammad):

Your cure is within you, yet you do not sense it;
Your sickness is from yourself, yet you do not see it.
You think that you are an insignificant speck;
But within you is enfolded the greatest cosmos.
So you are 'the clear Book',
By whose letters the hidden becomes manifest.

The cure we are seeking is within our heart – but our outer senses cannot comprehend this, limited as they are to impressions made by objects of this world. It is only our Spirit, when awakened by the quest for the reality of beauty, that will help us to 'see' the deeper dimensions of reality. It will help us to glimpse, not with our eyes, but by the 'eye' of the heart, what the Prophet of Islam meant in the following saying – one of the most mysterious teachings of Islamic spirituality. According to the Prophet, God says:

My earth cannot contain Me.
My Heaven cannot contain Me.
But the heart of my faithful servant does contain Me.

Having an intuition of the unfathomable depths of one's own heart: that is the beginning of the quest for the reality of beauty. Once found, beauty provides the cure for every ailment – and gives infinitely more than one can imagine. And what beauty can do for one soul, it can do for all souls. To learn the importance of value and values, both at the level of the individual and at the level of society, is imperative. This can only be appreciated through a heartfelt desire. Not only must there be an intuition, but this must be preceded by a desire to understand both oneself and, through oneself, the hearts of others.

Beauty shall save the world.

CHAPTER THREE

The Middle (Training)

Training in medicine is a process that begins while a medical student, and continues for the rest of one's medical life, after qualification. It is, of course, continually punctuated by exams.

One of the best things I realised was the benefit of laughter in the practice of medicine. This was made a lot easier by the wonderful book by Samuel Shem, *The House of God*, which was a parody of medical training. It made the intensity of medical training a lot more bearable, but it had its practical uses. One of the anecdotes I remember most, and was able to put into practice, was a situation where I was the house officer on call for the casualty department. This was at Northwick Park Hospital, where every now and then vagrants would come in essentially to spend the night in the hospital, as it was either too cold to sleep outside or they could not be bothered to visit any shelter to which they were attached. This meant that the patient, once they came in, usually drunk, had to be assessed. Since their clothes and bodies were often significantly infested with lice, clothes had to be cut off and the patient had to be washed down in a special room prior to being given a bed for the night. On one such occasion, I had already admitted several acutely unwell patients suffering from heart attacks and strokes, and was just on my way to bed at approximately 3 a.m. when I was called to assess a vagrant. Having recently encountered this scenario in Shem's book, I had the bright idea of offering the vagrant £5 if he went down the road to St Mary's Hospital, where I assured him he would enjoy a better night's sleep. He accepted my money gratefully and left.

Medical training is by far the most interactive apprenticeship. It demands interaction with human beings at their most vulnerable. It requires deep empathy, the ability to see the other as oneself, which goes beyond systematic analysis in its essence, but at the same time presupposes discernment, reason and judgement.

This apprenticeship, pre-qualification, takes approximately three years in the UK and approximately two years in the US. It involves a traditional approach, with an assignment to the various different disciplines of medicine and a comprehensive exposition of all aspects of medical practice. Post-qualification, one spends from five to eight years leading to a specialisation. Thereafter, one may also do a fellowship for one to two years, leading to a subspecialisation.

It involves first of all a mastery of the process of taking a history. This art is a formal and systematic approach to eliciting a constellation of symptoms from an individual, even a child, as comprehensively as possible. Each symptom (or complaint) is dealt with specifically and broken down into components. These are then cross-referenced to a whole series of other symptoms that may or may not be related to the original symptom or symptoms (or complaint or complaints). This, together with a detailed previous medical history, and a fairly comprehensive social history to understand the context in which these new complaints have arisen, leads to a probable diagnosis or a set of diagnoses, which in turn forms a hypothesis. Although this, to some extent, uses the faculty of reason to analyse the constellation of symptoms that have been presented, it also requires the process of memory to try and match it to other symptoms you have either read about or know about, that may present in this way. But then comes intuition, in many ways the most important element: the provisional diagnosis arrived at is an intuitive hypothesis, and most often requires a high degree of imagination to 'see' and then formulate a hypothetical cause of the illness. We have an interplay between reason, imagination, intuition and memory. Only once a comprehensive history has been taken, and a range of possibilities are arrayed in the mind, can the process of examination begin.

The examination is both objective and subjective. It is objective in that it is comprehensive, but it is subjective in that it is used as a means of either confirming or refuting a series of hypotheses. It is very much in the realm of reason and the dialectic. A history alone will lead to a diagnosis in approximately 70 per cent of patients, but an important further 20 per cent can only be crystallised once an examination has been performed. The examination has to be systematic and thorough. So, investigations only add 10% to make a diagnosis but are also useful in either confirming or refuting a diagnosis.

I recall my second year of training following qualification as a doctor, when I worked for Professor Lindsay Symon at the National Hospital for Neurology and Neurosurgery, Queen's Square. On my first day as his senior house officer (or SHO), I learnt something that was to be of tremendous value to me for the rest of my medical life. At that time, I was on call at the hospital every other night. Many nights involved the admission of patients as emergencies. I would have to start the ward round with Professor Symon at seven o'clock in the morning, but every other day, when I was on call, I was also obliged to call in at nine o'clock at night to discuss his patients. I still remember the first night I called him. I had been round to see his patients and reported in to say that the patients were well.

'Very good, dear boy,' he replied, 'but have you examined Mrs so-and-so's visual fields?'

Of course, I hadn't. I didn't think it was necessary to do so, because her problem was with her lower limbs. She had a neurological issue that emanated from the spine, on which Professor Symon had just operated. As to what this had to do with her visual fields, I didn't know then and still don't to this day.

'No, Professor, I haven't,' I admitted.

'Ah. If I were you, dear boy, I would do so.' He promptly put down the phone.

I rushed upstairs to the recovery room and theatres, examined the patient's visual fields, which, as expected, were totally normal, and went back downstairs. I rang him with the good news.

'That's very good, dear boy, but what about Mr so-and-so's ankle reflexes?'

I had not examined Mr so-and-so's ankle reflexes because his operation had been for a trapped nerve in his hand (carpal tunnel syndrome), and I couldn't see what that had to do with his ankle reflexes. Nevertheless, I duly rushed back upstairs and tested his ankle reflexes. Then, after a moment of reflection, I performed a full neurological examination on every one of Professor Symon's patients. This took quite a while. I think he knew it.

I went back downstairs, called him, and told him that Mr so-and-so's ankle reflexes were intact.

'Excellent, dear boy. Goodnight!' The line went dead.

After that night, and for the whole six months I was there, every other day when I was on call, except for the two weeks that I was on vacation, I examined every single patient comprehensively, regardless of complaint.

At the end of my six months, Professor Symon gave me some book tokens (an honour, which I am told was an extremely rare occurrence) to thank me for looking after his private patients, and asked if I had ever thought about a career in neurosurgery. I replied that I hadn't, and I was instead considering becoming an orthopaedic surgeon, because 90 per cent of the patients that we treated, be they knee replacement, hip replacement or post-traumatic patients, left the ward better than when they were admitted. I told him in the humblest possible way that I'd seen only approximately 10 per cent of patients admitted to a neurosurgery brain unit leave the wards either the same or better than when they arrived. I asked him how he had come to terms with this. He paused, then said,

'Ah, dear boy, one must only think about one's successful outcomes. I am afraid in my line of work, a poor outcome in terms of function is the sacrifice one has to make, for example, when one removes a brain tumour. One must always think about the fact that the benefits are better than what were to happen if the operation did not occur. One must never immerse oneself in a bad outcome, be it inevitable or not. To do so would leave you like my predecessor, who at the end of his career was incapable of holding a knife.'

Again, an incredibly salutary lesson.

I recall doing the same post as a young neurosurgical trainee (or SHO) at Queen's Square and accepting a patient from St Thomas'. She was a forty-year-old solicitor who had suffered a massive stroke due to a brain haemorrhage, which my senior registrar, Charlie Marks, who was a wonderful trainer and a sanguine human being, treated promptly and stopped her getting worse. Nevertheless, she was left with a severe paralysis of half her body, including the need to be tube fed.

A few days later I was called by the staff at St Thomas', who wanted to know how she was getting on. I responded to them cheerfully that she was getting on 'very well' and that I would keep them abreast of her progress. I still remember Charlie overhearing my conversation.

'So,' he said to me, 'your definition of "very well" is a patient who has half her face and body paralysed, who needs a tube to be fed and who is drooling from her mouth? What you mean by "very well" is that she is alive.' Again, a poignant reminder of the limitations of medical practice and about understanding disability.

• • •

The Pavlovian nature of my initial training was exemplified by my having to hold the crash bleep after I had finished my house jobs. Those involved in the crash team would rush to any cardiac arrest to try to revive the patient who had crashed, and this could occur at any time, sometimes while we were asleep – we would often still be getting dressed on our sprint to the crash site. I recall being on vacation at home and hearing an alarm going off next door in my sister's room early one morning, and rushing down the stairs, getting dressed in the process. I was met by my alarmed mother, who didn't quite understand what I was doing at that hour, half naked and running down the stairs!

• • •

After I had completed my senior house officer training and my registrar training, I began to attend interviews. One of the jobs I applied for was that of a senior registrar at the Royal National Orthopaedic Hospital in London. Unsurprisingly, the chairman of the interview committee was none other than Professor George Bentley, who had failed me in my Orthopaedic Assessment clinical exam when I was a student – which, ultimately, was how I ended up choosing orthopaedics as my speciality. I sat at the foot of the table. There were nearly twenty surgeons present, all from the hospitals linked to the training at the Royal National Orthopaedic Hospital. They systematically interviewed me, and then finally it was Professor Bentley's turn. He asked me how it was that I had become interested in orthopaedics. I told him. I got the job.

The most remarkable thing about training, as it was then, was the intense number of hours and the pressure under which one trained. The other astonishing thing was the breadth of training, in that before one could train as an orthopaedic surgeon, one had to spend at least a year as a registrar in general surgery. This is no longer required.

During the process of training (other than being a medical student, and even sometimes at the medical student stage), the extent to which one performed procedures was remarkable. As an SHO (during my third year of post-qualification training), I would have performed several hernia operations and appendectomies, all under scrupulous supervision by competent colleagues, and then, as an orthopaedic registrar (a trainee typically in their fourth or fifth year of specialist training, or about seventh or eighth years of training post-qualification), hip replacements, knee replacements, over a hundred femoral nails for broken femurs, over a hundred tibial nails for broken tibias, and so on. By the end of my training (approximately seven years from the time I became an SHO – approximately seven years post-qualification – to the time I became a consultant/senior lecturer), I would have seen, at an intense level, many surgical specialities including neurosurgery and general surgery, which in those days included abdominal surgery, surgery for aortic aneurysms, for veins, colorectal surgery and, of course, orthopaedics. I must say that by the time I became a consultant there was little that would terrify me in my chosen speciality, particularly because I had such a comprehensive knowledge of the rest of the body.

Thereafter, rather than employing an 'approach' surgeon (as in the US), I did most of my own abdominal or neck approaches for surgery to the spine in those particular areas, meaning that I would be comfortable, for example, around the neck, dissecting out the spine around the oesophagus, trachea, larynx etc. The same was true of the abdomen, where I would have no difficulty in preserving and operating around the lungs, the large arteries, the veins, and abdominal contents including the liver, spleen, etc. I am delighted to say that in all my years as a consultant, and having taken many of these approaches, I have never had any major problems with any of them. That is a testament not to my skill but to my comprehensive and excellent training.

The European Working Time Directive has, in my opinion, done a great disservice to medical training, although it was for many years exempt, and only brought in at the request of some highly politically ambitious junior doctors, who threw the baby of their greatest asset – their remarkable training – out with the bathwater of their antisocial hours.

The process of examinations, as alluded to previously, encompasses both theory and practice. It is impossible to pass an exam without competence both in the written side of the exams, covering all aspects of the speciality, followed by a clinical examination involving long, comprehensive histories and examinations of the patient, followed by short cases where one would look at a patient for a brief period of time and, based on the external appearances, come up with a provisional or formal diagnosis.

I recall when I was an orthopaedic trainee at the Royal National Orthopaedic Hospital, George Bentley used to do the rounds with us, and teach us using the various patients on the ward. He would insist on us turning up on a Saturday, even though we were never paid for this. Those of us who took the exam – and even those who were taking the exam, but from other hospitals – would attend these rounds, and we would all work together to systematically cover the whole of orthopaedics before our final inset examination. These exams were held twice a year. An order of merit was established across the whole year, and the top trainee of the year – based on his performance in the Intercollegiate FRCS Orthopaedic Exams carried out across Ireland, Wales, England and Scotland – would receive the Walter Mercer Gold Medal from the President of the Royal College of Surgeons of whichever of the countries where he or she had obtained the initial Fellowship Certificate. I won the Walter Mercer Gold Medal, which I value to this day. It was a privilege to work under the tutelage of George Bentley and all my trainers, who were systematic and comprehensive in teaching me both the art and the practice of medicine in general, and orthopaedics in particular.

Training was a continuing effort. It started as a medical student but the initial exam – MBBS or BM BCh in Oxford or the MB BChir in Cambridge or MD in the US – was simply a milestone in the whole process of education, which then continues for the rest of your practising life, each milestone – whether it be as a senior house officer, registrar, senior registrar or consultant – being simply stepping off one ladder to start on another one. To end one exam is to begin another!

Prior to taking up my post as a consultant, I did many short fellowships in the US. I greatly enjoyed this, not least because it allowed me to explore that beautiful and still virgin country by Greyhound bus. An interesting anecdote is my application to be a fellow at the Harborview Medical Center in Seattle, affiliated to the Swedish Hospital. I was amazed to be accepted immediately. My physical arrival, however, was not greeted with a great deal of enthusiasm. Surprised, I discussed this with a Scandinavian friend then resident in New York, whom I visited on the first weekend of my fellowship. He told me, to my amazement, that the Swedish Hospital and Harborview positively discriminated in favour of individuals of Scandinavian origin. It made some sense. My bosses, Ted Hanson, Berniscke, Jens Chapman and Swintkowski, were all Scandinavian. Also my name – N-o-r-d-e-e-n, as it was spelt there – was, it seems, the most common name in the Scandinavian phonebook. Imagine their surprise at seeing me in the flesh! I had my opportunity to explain. While assisting during a complex operation, I was casually asked about my origins. I earnestly explained, to pin-drop silence, that my family were the descendants of a Viking boat that had been stranded off the coast of Sri Lanka. This was greeted with some incredulity and then laughter as they began to understand the joke. The rest of my stay was most educational, and very pleasant.

It is not surprising that medical students and doctors tend to marry other doctors. Few can understand or put up with the demands of medical life. As a doctor, it is difficult not to see life in terms of diseases. It is imperative in these circumstances always to have some sort of external hobby or an individual with whom one spends one's time, whether it be family or friend, who takes you away from your practice so that you can look at it both objectively and subjectively. To understand what disease is, one needs as reference every walk of life.

* * *

There is then the question of research. This is the culpable area in terms of creeping darkness. Given the way in which research is funded in the UK, it has become a citadel of undertaking research for the sake of being seen to be doing something. Grant committees are populated by the same academics who come from the universities. Being academics, they prefer to award grants to other academics. This may be simple speculation, but there is always a feeling around grant committees that it is Buggins' turn.

On the face of it, this might seem a reasonable thing to do, but given the great deal of research that occurs, a large number of animals are perhaps being caused unnecessary pain or being bred for experimentation and ultimate death.

To be clear, I am not a vegetarian, although I would be quite happy being one. I don't want to get into the politics of animal research or indeed hunting, but I do not think it is unreasonable to feel that when one is undertaking the culling of animals for research or for sport, one should try to restrict any suffering to the minimum possible, and indeed limit the animals killed for these purposes to as small a number as possible. It is my personal preference not to undertake the sacrifice of an animal for these purposes, although I think it is entirely reasonable to take the life of an animal for the purpose of food.

The purpose of research is to carry out an experiment or a series of experiments to either confirm or refute a hypothesis. In doing so, one has to be mindful of the absolute need for doing research for research's sake. Many animals suffer and die when it may be possible to find an alternative way of answering the same questions. One has to be mindful of taking the life of an animal in the name of research. Vivisection is something not to be undertaken with impunity.

There is no doubt that the ability to conduct research systematically is something to be greatly admired and valued, but again an example of means becoming an end is that of fraudulent research, undertaken purely to build up a portfolio or CV. There have been too many recent examples of this.

* * *

Training and conversation are the keystones to a career in medicine. Training needs to be preserved, deepened, calibrated, maintained and nurtured. This is achieved by none other than the art of conversation. Conversations are best conducted not in front of a screen of one sort or another, but face to face, which, thank goodness, is still the case in the practice of training. However, again we are at risk of teleconferences and Skype calls taking over. These can become isolating.

It is important to put everything in its place, to put everything in context, to have a proper sense of perspective. To have context and perspective, it is necessary to have a vision. To have a vision, it is important to see the different dimensions we inhabit. Our planet, in the context of the universe. Ourselves, in the context of the planet. The importance of the planet and the importance of ourselves. The importance of ourselves in the context of the importance of all other selves. We need to nurture a holistic vision of the universe, one in which each and every soul is connected organically and spiritually to every other soul.

It is reassuring that medicine still maintains the integral art of conversation, when it is itself understood as an art; but alas, the art of conversation is becoming marginalised by those who see medicine only as a science. It is difficult to give the art of conversation its due when one is increasingly faced with time constraints. The sudden revelation of an ailment will require much longer than the ten minutes or so available for a consultation. It is, however, possible through the art of conversation to get to the core of the problem. This is a skill that is both an art and a science. We know that healing a patient presupposes a correct understanding of the cause of the illness. We may well be able to use our instruments to measure certain symptoms and arrive at an accurate diagnosis of the physical cause of the illness. But with what instruments do we measure the psychological and emotional aspects of the illness?

We have no instrument other than the spiritual science, or the medical art, of empathy, of intuitively feeling what the patient is experiencing, on the emotional level as well as the physical level. And without conversation, without engaging with the whole person sitting in front of us, we are not going to come close to intuiting the deeper causes of illness afflicting the patient, let alone transmit to the patient the empathy of understanding, the love and the kindness that may turn out to be a far more efficacious means of curing the illness than any pill. In medical training, what must therefore be preserved and deepened – and, I would argue, enriched by the insights of the psychology and the spiritual traditions of healing – is the art of conversation between the seasoned master and the inexperienced apprentice.

CHAPTER FOUR

The End (Practice)

In this last of meeting places
We grope together
And avoid speech
Gathered on this beach of the tumid river
'The Hollow Men' by T.S. Eliot

S.W.R.D. Bandaranaike, the first prime minister of Sri Lanka and a former secretary of the Oxford Union, assassinated in his prime allegedly for a misuse of power, wrote: 'Often when power is sought as a means to an end, the means becomes the end.' So it is with medicine. Few go into medicine with anything other than the best intention. The intention of becoming part of the process and culture of compassionate care. The way in which the structure works makes it easy for a paradigm of command and control to take over, as the currency within this system is one based on power.

A darkness has descended into the practice of medicine because the culture of care that used to exist within medicine has been replaced by a culture of command and control. The culture of care has been destroyed by the culture of command and control. This is no different in the US, although the drivers are different. In the UK, the currency is institutional power based on hierarchy. In the US, it is money. Cost and reimbursement. But managers are managers wherever they may be. What follows is applicable not only in the UK and the US, but in any healthcare system.

The National Health Service has a series of divisions and subdivisions. The senior management, whose pay grades are based on seniority and service, oversee the NHS as a whole. Beneath them comes a division between commissioners – those who commission services (funded by the government) – and the providers of services, who can be broadly separated into general practitioners and the hospitals (or trusts). General practitioners have their own management structure to help manage the doctors, and similarly, hospitals have their own management system to help manage the hospital staff.

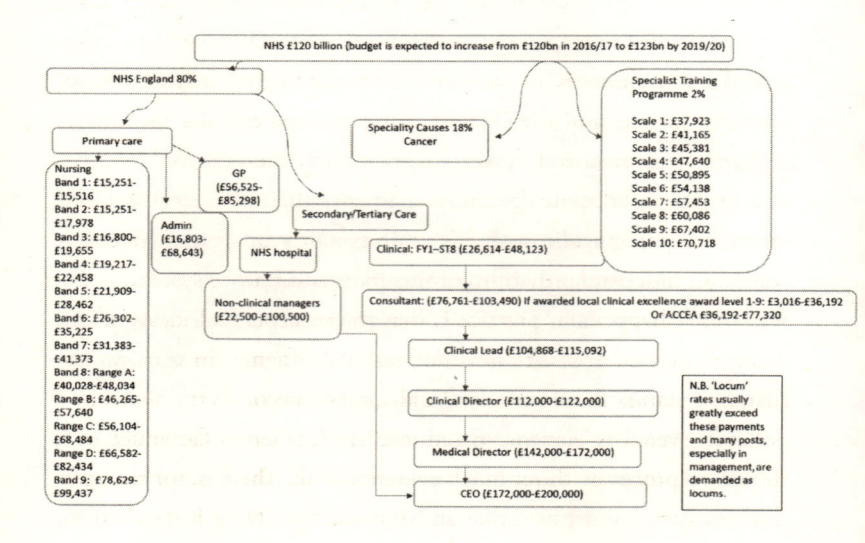

NHS £120 billion (budget is expected to increase from £120bn in 2016/17 to £123bn by 2019/20)

NHS England 80%

Specialist Training Programme 2%

Speciality Causes 18% Cancer

Scale 1: £37,923
Scale 2: £41,165
Scale 3: £45,381
Scale 4: £47,640
Scale 5: £50,895
Scale 6: £54,138
Scale 7: £57,453
Scale 8: £60,086
Scale 9: £67,402
Scale 10: £70,718

Primary care

Nursing
Band 1: £15,251-£15,516
Band 2: £15,251-£17,978
Band 3: £16,800-£19,655
Band 4: £19,217-£22,458
Band 5: £21,909-£28,462
Band 6: £26,302-£35,225
Band 7: £31,383-£41,373
Band 8: Range A: £40,028-£48,034
Range B: £46,265-£57,640
Range C: £56,104-£68,484
Range D: £66,582-£82,434
Band 9: £78,629-£99,437

GP (£56,525-£85,298)

Admin (£16,803-£68,643)

Secondary/Tertiary Care

NHS hospital

Non-clinical managers (£22,500-£100,500)

Clinical: FY1–ST8 (£26,614-£48,123)

Consultant: (£76,761-£103,490) If awarded local clinical excellence award level 1-9: £3,016-£36,192 Or ACCEA £36,192-£77,320

Clinical Lead (£104,868-£115,092)

Clinical Director (£112,000-£122,000)

Medical Director (£142,000-£172,000)

CEO (£172,000-£200,000)

N.B. 'Locum' rates usually greatly exceed these payments and many posts, especially in management, are demanded as locums.

There is a subtle difference. General practices are run and managed by principals, effectively senior general practitioners, who have ownership of the practices and the way in which they are run. They are on the whole self-governing, but there are still salaried general practitioners, particularly in rural areas, who are funded directly by the National Health Service. Hospitals are run and managed by professional managers. Hospital managers and doctors are employees of the hospital, and do have a significant say in the running of the hospital, but on the whole hospitals are run by a Chief Executive Officer, a Chief Operational Officer, a Chief Financial Officer and a Medical Director, who is the head of the hierarchy of the hospital medical staff.

Both structures are funded by the government. Both structures, both clinical and management, have a pay scale based on designation and seniority. For GPs, you have GP trainees who are paid according to their years of service, and then GP principals or general practitioners who have not only a salary but also the ability to have a share of the practice management itself. In hospitals, clinicians are designated into trainees, who again are paid according to their number of years of service, and who have in the past been called senior house officers (registrars and fellows), and then consultants. The hospitals also have associate specialists who have their own structure and again are paid in terms of their number of years' experience, but function independently of the consultant and trainee system.

What happens in practice is that the precepts and ideals of this 'culture of care' translate into dogma. This dogma, in turn, in the name of 'standardisation of care' and 'targets', becomes translated into what is revered as 'evidence-based medicine', when in fact much of it is really a process without much evidence at all. There is, for example, little evidence to support that an 'appraisal' (appraisal is required for every doctor examining every aspect of their practice) and 'revalidation' (required every 5 years including patient and colleague feedback) do any good. A process of appraisal that occurs for every practising doctor means that one has to be signed off by an appraisee, and this goes through a whole series of time-consuming processes both for the appraiser and the appraisee. This eventually becomes a box-ticking exercise that would occupy a significant amount of time on behalf of both individuals, and yet there is little evidence to back it.

Now we also have, on top of the traditional training of ward rounds and clinic appointments, a process called an MDT (Multi-Disciplinary Team) meeting. This involves a number of practitioners, including nursing staff, physiotherapists, occupational therapists, surgeons and anaesthetists, all of whom are making decisions on behalf of the patient (or 'client', as they are known). In many hospitals, the only individual excluded from the process is the patient.

These meetings are now key to medical practice. Nothing can be done without a meeting, at least in the hospital setting. It is conducted as a means of justifying treatment (therapy). The treatment is now the star turn, not the patient.

Traditionally, at least when I was a registrar at the Middlesex Hospital, these meetings actively involved the patients, who had the opportunity to be examined in front of the clinicians, by doctors in training, and whenever an examination was incomplete, a full examination was insisted on by their assembled peers. At the end of this process, the patient would have the ability to ask questions of all those in the meeting. The modern MDT excludes the most important individual: the patient. Again, the decision is made on behalf of the patient and the outcome of the meeting is communicated to the patient, often simply by letter but sometimes verbally.

The outcome of the meeting would usually involve a 'standard of care'. Anyone delivering care outside this standard would be deemed an 'outlier'. For example, I undertake most of my approaches to the abdomen and have done so safely for over twenty years, and I was told recently that if I continued to do so, I too would be considered an outlier. I have therefore to employ an 'approach surgeon' to make the spine visible to me, having made the incision and the approach to the spine. In fact, in private practice, often the approach surgeons are paid more than I am. From my point of view, I would be paid no differently whether I did the approach or not, so why not simply get the approach surgeon in and have as many cups of coffee as it takes until the approach surgeon has exposed the spine for me? I suspect that this reflects the training of the more recent spinal surgeons, who have no general surgical training and who would be uncomfortable in doing their own exposures. This is the cost of increasing specialisation.

* * *

There is no longer a general surgeon. There is now a liver specialist, a kidney specialist, or in orthopaedics, a foot and ankle specialist, a shoulder specialist, a knee specialist, a hip specialist, a spine specialist, and so on. Worse still, many hospitals no longer assign a patient to a particular surgeon. In any event, patients are now 'owned' not by a consultant as they used to be in the past, but by the hospital or trust, so whenever one has a conversation, the trust, which indemnifies everyone, is the only entity not in the room. So the trust takes ownership of the patient and indemnifies the individual consultant. Often the patient will be seen by different consultants, whereas in the past the patients belonged to the consultant's 'firm' and the treatment administered would be by members of this firm, including the consultant, the registrar, the senior house officer and the houseman. Now, the patient would be seen in clinic by one individual consultant. We have a consultant-led service and many of the consultants are, as I alluded to before, trained only in their speciality and would not have an overview of the speciality, never mind the whole of medicine. The patient would then most likely be operated on by another consultant, and be followed up on different occasions by different consultants. This is hardly continuity of care, or indeed a culture of care, let alone compassionate care. Thus, the doctor–patient relationship – which to the 'trust' is probably an undesirable element – is gradually eroded and there enters now a patient–trust relationship. There is thus a diminution of the responsibility that each consultant felt or has felt in the past.

* * *

To this comes a culture of blame. If anything in the treatment of a patient is not satisfactory, if it simply means a poor outcome, someone has to be blamed. This engenders a focus on outcomes, simply to apportion blame, whether it be medico-legally or whether it is used as a weapon in the internecine warfare that goes on between individuals and departments in a trust. When I briefly headed my trust's litigation directive, I examined the cases that were in open litigation and found out that some, but not all, had an RCA (Root Cause Analysis) associated with them. An RCA is a systematic investigation of a process that involves a critical incident, which is either a near incident, a close shave or for any other reason. It may also include a complaint of poor outcome. This laborious process then produces a report that is usually a means of apportioning blame, often arbitrarily.

It is accepted that when there is an avoidable incident, it is usually a systemic failure. In other words, when things go wrong, it is never one thing or process that is responsible. It is usually a whole series of failings or shortcomings – i.e., 'the system'. These RCAs, or inquiries, exist simply to reflect the fact that every aspect of a process needs to be examined, and the purpose of this is not to apportion blame but to ensure that whatever failure there was in the whole process or 'care pathway' would be rectified, and that this failure would be avoided in future.

I found that only approximately 5 per cent of incidents that went on to litigation ever had an RCA conducted as part of them. The majority of RCAs that were conducted seemed whimsical, to apportion blame and thus intimidate the individual or individuals concerned. An example of this is the Francis Report on the failings of care at the Mid Staffordshire NHS Foundation Trust, published in 2013, which concluded that a culture of command and control has replaced the culture of care that used to exist within the NHS.

* * *

As training has become more singular and process-driven, so has the approach to patient care, which, as we have discussed, is now a dogma based on a whole series of measurements, rather than any ability to use the faculties of imagination or intuition. These have all become algorithm-driven. If one were to use intuition, imagination, or in fact any form of initiative, then there is always the fear that one will be classified as an outlier, subject to sanction. This fear, underpinned by the various sanctions that have been put in place by a now rigidly established management, ensures that not only is a culture of command and control in place, but with it a culture of fear. A fear of being an outlier, a fear of an inquiry, a fear of an investigation and a fear of a sanction that might then go into your record. A fear of losing your job. Gone is the ability to nurture a trainee on a firm. Gone is the chain of responsibility, and the responsibility that goes with it. This has now been replaced by numerous managers as enforcers of processes and algorithms.

* * *

There are more managers than beds in the National Health Service. The NHS has the third highest number of employees in the world, behind the Chinese army and the Indian railway system. Seventy per cent of NHS costs goes on salaries. Managers have their own structure, their own courses, and operate independently of the clinical framework.

When I first started as a consultant, my hospital was run by a medical director and chief nurse. The management was effectively individuals who were there to execute, prosecute and implement the decisions made by the medical director and the chief nurse. It worked well, and was extremely efficient. Then came successive governments, who swelled management numbers as a job creation scheme, to stem the three million unemployment rate. What these governments did not take into account – or they might have, but chose to ignore – were the future costs to the taxpayer, and thus to future generations, of the burden of so many new 'final salary pension schemes'.

Managers now go on courses on how to deal with 'difficult doctors'. They have algorithms as to how to deal with doctors who are not compliant. I do not know of a single course where doctors are taught to deal with difficult managers. Doctors are taught how to be managers but never how to manage managers. I know of at least one young clinician with a potentially good practice as a clinician who has altered his life and goals to enter into the management structure, to reach the top of the management ladder, and to end up as chief executive officer of a hospital. It is rare that they spend more than a few years there, as they tend to flit from one chief executive post to another. There is no continuity of management.

Those of us who are left at the hospital have to provide continuity of care. This is despite being in a system that is increasingly over-managed, where change is enforced simply for the sake of enforcing change. Once again, the means has become the end.

The result of any treatment has always to be a combination of both expectation and outcome. There has been no measure and no initiative whatsoever to deal with expectation. Expectation at its worst will become entitlement. What a patient expects out of an operation or treatment, and what the best outcome might be, are often two different things. There is neither subjective nor objective measure of what is expected. This can have disastrous consequences.

There was a recent litigation in which a patient had a poor outcome after spinal surgery – a simple discectomy, I believe. The treating surgeon had quoted to her an 85 per cent chance of a good outcome. The claimant's expert said that the chances were more in the order of approximately 80 per cent. The claimant won the case on the basis that the defending surgeon had inflated the chances of success. There has to be a systematic effort:

1. To understand expectation.
2. For a patient to clearly communicate what this expectation is.
3. To provide a means of managing this expectation.

This surely is the first step.

There has been a huge emphasis on outcomes. This is akin to the debacle that has been going on for quite a while, given the commissioner/provider split that exists between the hospital and those who commission the services at the hospital. The whole thrust of the funding of the NHS has been focused on how services are commissioned. Commissioning groups, special commissioning groups, GP consultants etc, have all been formed to manage commissioning, which is effectively a way of rationing or limiting the money spent on the provision of a service. Commissioners act as a gatekeeper to the funds that go to paying the providers, i.e. the hospital. Very little has been done until recently about how hospitals should be reimbursed or how much they should be reimbursed, hence an increasing focus on standardisation of care. To this end, there has been a huge focus on 'outcomes'. However, to focus on the commissioning services without any deep analysis on the provision of services is as poor as to focus on 'outcomes' without paying any attention to expectation.

My friend and colleague Professor Tim Briggs CBE was so moved by the Francis Report that he undertook the publication of a report entitled 'Getting It Right First Time' (GIRFT). Following the publication of the Francis Report in 2013, there was a further examination of an additional six thousand deaths at fourteen other hospitals. Briggs was deeply troubled by the evidence of poor care that emerged. He concluded that in the previous fifteen years, the main drivers in the NHS had been financial performance and a culture driven by targets. Front-line clinicians had been slowly marginalised and, in many cases, had lost any influence or shaping of the hospital's agenda. The failings that occurred at Stafford Hospital occurred because the decision-making process was controlled by managers. There was a failure to understand the complexities of clinical care or the impact of one policy on another component of clinical care. There were no checks of this process by either the medical director or the chief nurse – or if there were, these individuals were already part of the management culture. Francis concluded that a command and control style crushed the culture of care in the NHS. This has led to a loss of morale and disengagement by clinicians.

The biggest cost to staff salary has been made by reducing the number of experienced clinical staff and increasing and altering the ward nursing structure, making patients increasingly reliant on healthcare assistants who, although well meaning, are not clinically trained. It was only a matter of time before a tipping point was reached and patient care suffered. This coincided with the introduction of an eighteen-week target, in which patients were guaranteed their treatment within a tight time frame, meaning that more and more patients were pushed into a system that was already close to breaking point. No clinician was surprised at these findings, which is shocking. It was Tim Briggs' view that senior clinicians must remain in roles with presence both on the clinical front line and on the ward, to improve the standard of care provided to patients and the trust. For example, a simple marker of the quality of care within a trust is the incidence of bed sores, which are highly preventable. In many instances, the available statistics are ignored.

The lifespan of a trust's chief executive is on average less than two years. There seems to be a complete loss of focus on the reason the boards are there, which should surely be to provide excellent and high-quality care for patients.

There is a complete lack of accountability. This is both from a clinical point of view and from a managerial point of view. Maintaining and improving current service levels can only be achieved if we accept that change is essential. A focus on commissioning of care will eventually directly influence how we provide care in hospital, which accounts for 70 per cent of the cost of the NHS.

* * *

Briggs was fundamentally of the belief that improvement could be achieved by fully engaging front-line commissioners to rework and reconfigure services while maintaining high-quality treatment. In his view, this would require a real shift in influence of clinical decision-making, with the managers backing the clinicians and joining up ownership of issues threatening both the quality of care and a sustainable financial position. A clinician-led management body would also ensure that management stood shoulder to shoulder with clinicians, to enable clinicians to do their job to a high standard and also attain financial sustainability.

This would have the effect of re-energising front-line commissions but would require tremendous leadership.

One way of accomplishing this, at least in orthopaedics, is to avoid the revision surgery that is required, as this surgery is both expensive and time-consuming. Infection is a demonstrated complication in patients, and 30 per cent of all revision surgery is affected by infection. If the infection rate, which currently varies from 1 to 4 per cent between hospitals, could be reduced to 0.2 per cent, as achieved at the Royal National Orthopaedic Hospital, this could save the NHS £300 million per annum, with a cumulative saving of £1.5 billion over five years.

Briggs also looked at litigation in orthopaedics, and found that the four commonest causes of orthopaedic litigation were all potentially preventable. He felt that both changes in practice and greater integration of services needed to occur to ensure timely and high-quality care for patients, which in his view would deliver the financial saving that had to be made.

Litigation within the Health Service is imperative and nowhere more so than in the delivery of medical care. This too is open to abuse and occurs particularly if there is a system that funds a litigant and their representatives, without holding a litigant to account. The way in which the current system operates ensures that a litigant can bring a claim that is funded by the state, and however weak or spurious the case may be, it will nevertheless reach a stage where, having determined that the case is weak or spurious, both the litigant and the litigant's representative (usually lawyers) are paid. This does not amount to accountability, and remains a strong incentive. We then have to have a system that either:

1. awards patients 'no fault' compensation, which I don't support, or
2. acknowledges litigation is in the best interest of justice.

I nevertheless feel that a balance has to be achieved where both a litigant and that their representative should be held to account in bringing forth and advancing litigation that has little chance of success. In this respect, litigants have now focused on a lack of consent in that:

a. potential alternatives to a particular form of treatment were not explained or discussed in depth;
b. the outcomes that were rehearsed (by which I mean the chances of success) were either knowingly or unknowingly exaggerated.

These have ended up in large claims and large awards, but there are numerous claims that never had any chance of success that nevertheless have been settled to the financial benefit of both litigants and lawyers. A balance has to be struck.

* * *

A real engagement between commissioners and providers and between clinicians and managers needs to be established, with all the stakeholders represented at every level. This can and must include patient advocates.

In addition, it is imperative that the management of expectations is also systematically undertaken, together with a clear understanding of likely outcomes. The only way to manage the ever rising cost of litigation is not only by improving outcomes but also by managing expectation.

• • •

So what can save the practice of medicine? Ultimately, both by empowering the patient (not to be defined as a 'client') and by a series of carers or doctors who are motivated first and foremost by a desire to heal, not those driven by financial incentives, or filled with managerial ambition, or terrified at the prospect of litigation. This would lead to the empowerment of the patient to take control of their pathway, to be involved at every stage of their care, to expect to be part of an MDT process, and to insist on named individuals being responsible for their care in a continuous manner – real human beings with whom they can engage and converse and from whom they can benefit, continuously and deeply, for the duration of their treatment.

This in turn requires empowerment of the caregiver, in terms of budget, appropriate time, appropriate resources and support from their organisation, to enable the clear identification of the doctor/patient relationship, expectation and outcome.

There are many sad examples in the lives of my colleagues where the means becomes an end. One of my senior colleagues was a distinguished orthopaedic surgeon dealing with children's foot deformities. He was incredibly dedicated to his patients, so much so that he would often spend his weekends at the hospital and sleep in, so that he could undertake operations.

We used to do ward rounds together, and end Friday afternoon in the pub with colleagues in different specialities. I was teetotal and therefore would not want to spend too much time in the pub, preferring to return home to my wife. There were three of us: my immediately senior colleague, my most senior colleague and me. I learnt subsequently that my colleague's dedication to his patients and his work led to a breakdown of his marriage and, ultimately, to divorce. It also led to problems with his children.

It always used to amuse me that many of my senior colleagues, who were surgeons, tended to marry their scrub nurse in theatre, usually as their second marriage. This was no doubt because they spent so much time together. However, what also used to amuse me was that, at regular intervals, they married younger versions of the same designation (i.e., a scrub nurse), and what was even more amusing was that they looked remarkably alike, simply younger.

The net result of this was that these individuals, despite having earned quite a tidy sum through their practice within the NHS and subsequently in private practice, and achieved a degree of wealth that included a large house and car, were hit progressively hard by the British divorce laws, so that by the end of their careers (and after their third or fourth marriage), they ended up in a bedsit. Meanwhile, their ex-wives retained the (successively smaller) houses they had occupied during their respective marriages.

What this shows us is that we must never allow ourselves to become unilateral, monolithic personalities. If we reduce ourselves to being one-dimensional – even if that one dimension is medical care and the successful cure of a particular physical ailment – then we cannot be true to our immortal personality, 'made in the image of God', as the Book of Genesis tells us. The Prophet Muhammad tells us the same thing, but also reminds us of the absolute, infinite perfection in whose image we are made: 'Truly, God is beautiful and He loves Beauty.' If we wish to be true to that beauty, and we wish to manifest our love of all things beautiful, we have to reflect that beauty in our own lives. Beauty implies perfect harmony, and harmony implies a diversity of elements brought together in a pleasing whole. When we allow one part of our being to split off from the rest, there is disharmony and thus, eventually, the hidden ugliness of an obsessive personality: a brilliant surgeon dying alone, in self-imposed exile from his family.

All of us in the medical profession need to take much more seriously the proverb cited by Jesus: 'Physician, heal thyself'. The only way in which the physician can heal himself is to go from physics (which means simply 'nature' in Greek) to metaphysics (which means 'beyond nature'), to go from the material to the spiritual, and to understand that our material dimension – our bodily health – is more dependent upon the spiritual state of our soul than our scientific instruments can possibly measure. To heal ourselves, we need to realise that our fragmented state of soul must become once again whole, reflecting the beauty in whose image we are made. As my late and great teacher Dr Martin Lings explains:

> *To be perfectly well, the soul must be complete. 'Holiness', 'wholeness' and 'health' are in origin the same word, and have merely been differentiated in form, and in meaning, through the fragmentation of language. The virtues of sincerity and simplicity are inseparable from this perfection, for each in its own way means undividedness of soul.*

He continues thus, giving us an answer to the question we might pose: how can beauty help us to attain this health, wholeness and holiness?

> *The purpose of religion as a whole is to knit together all looseness in man by setting up in his soul an impetus towards the centre which will bring it once more within range of the attraction of the Heart; and if this applies above all to religious rites, it is*

true of everything that has a spiritual function. For example, when we contemplate a work of truly sacred art, the whole soul comes together as if in answer to an imperative summons. There is no question of any fragmentary reaction, for we cannot marvel enough. Here lies the essence of a sacred civilization.

CHAPTER FIVE

An Epidemic of Harm

There has been an epidemic of harm in the medical universe. An epidemic that flies in the face of the first precept of medical practice: 'Do no harm'. This has caught us unawares.

The number of deaths in the US from prescription and illicit opiate misuse rose fourfold between 1999 and 2015, and drug misuse is now the leading cause of death of Americans under the age of fifty. This over-prescribing continues today and must change to reduce the risk of subsequent inappropriate use. We have come to the stage where deaths are blamed on the failure to provide addiction treatment and on increasing inability to limit cheap street drugs with ever more synthetic, deadly opioids, such as fentanyl. Moralising and criminalising are merely sticking plasters to stem the tide of death and misery. To find a remedy requires identification of a cause.

In 2013 there were 250 million prescriptions for painkillers, enough for a bottle of pills for everyone. Even President Trump was sufficiently moved to declare the epidemic a national emergency. But there is no plan. The Centers for Disease Control and Prevention (CDC) has stated that drug misuse claimed more than 52,000 lives in the US in 2015, 33,000 of which followed an overdose of illicit opioids. The CDC also estimates that more than 300,000

Americans have been involved in the overdose of prescription opioids since the year 2000.

There have been various solutions suggested, including better access to medication-assisted treatment; ensuring the availability of the overdose rescue drug naloxone; enforcing existing legislation that compels insurers to cover substance use disorders (as they do physical disorders); and expanding access for inpatient mental health care for poor and disabled Americans. In addition, there is a great push for federal prosecutors to get tough on drug offences.

However, the rise in opioid prescribing has been blamed on economic decline and social fragmentation. The association between cause and effect – that of an increase in negative outcomes associated with opioid addition, including broken families, and overdose and drug-related threats – has emphasised a cure rather than prevention. A syringe-exchange programme, a special initiative to fund mental health and drug treatment, and even an anonymous surveillance programme have been set up to try to stem the problem, but most professionals agree that the programmes have been used as a means to perpetuate it. Most people come to centres such as these simply to get needles.

Overdoses from prescription opioids are now the driving factor in the increase in opioid overdose deaths, and, ironically, most states and counties are now filing lawsuits against drug makers for costs related to opioid misuse, alleging that their marketing positions downplay the risks and overplay the benefits of opioids for chronic non-cancer pain. There is an increasing recognition that this is a wound we will not be able to heal unless surgeons and other physicians change their behaviour.

There is an increasing focus on multimodal pain management, and it is startling that one in sixteen surgery patients becomes a chronic opioid user. After chronic pain specialists, surgeons have the highest rate of opioid prescribing in the US; however, 70 to 80 per cent of these (over)prescribed opioids are not used immediately after common surgical procedures. Instead, they are 'stockpiled' to be used as non-prescribed medication by patients or others in their household.

It comes as no surprise that the best approach to all of this is prevention. Agreed, the focus on prevention only can result in the marginalisation of drug users (and those who want to sell drugs). However, it is astonishing that it is thought that the crisis is a consequence of prohibitive legislation – a failure to understand that the reverse is the case and the legislation is, in fact, a direct consequence of the crisis!

Closer to home, the most recent annual assessment of health and social care by the Care Quality Commission provides a snapshot of the current state of medical practice in England. Clearly, services are at full stretch and struggling to maintain standards. There are variations between men's and women's services, with ongoing pressure on staff and a deterioration of quality. Adult social care is identified as being of particular concern, with a reduction in nursing home beds and the provision of domiciliary care and a huge increase in the number of older patients not receiving the help they need. Standards in many services are likely to fall further in the future.

Success is defined as improved care, with strong leadership, engaged staff cultures, empowered staff and shared vision, as well as an outward-looking approach. I would define the challenge as finding a sustainable solution, rather than focusing on funding. It is to recognise that much management and clinical time is spent reducing financial deficits and meeting targets, leading to the unintended emphasis on operational matters at the expense of work to transform care.

This still fails to identify the underlying cause of the malaise. To identify the cause is halfway to identifying a remedy.

How is beauty to remedy this horror? How is beauty to remedy the crisis that pervades all the way down to the very roots of our society, to the extent – at the individual level – of being existential?

* * *

I recall with great fondness my days as a registrar (a specialist in training) in the Low Back Pain Clinic run by three of my senior colleagues, Andrew Ransford, Michael Edgar and Ernie Kirwan, at University College Hospital, the Middlesex Hospital and the Royal National Orthopaedic Hospital. They were elemental in giving me an insight into the relationship between human psychology and physical health.

I always listened to Andrew's perspective in any given situation. Andrew Ransford was a tall ex-rugby player, who was responsible for appointing me and giving me my first break as a trainee at UCH. I recall that the interview was one-to-one, without any managers present, and he gave me the job based on my CV and his interview. He has been a source of support and inspiration ever since, and a mentor to many of my colleagues and contemporaries both in orthopaedics and in spinal surgery. The interviews are much more formal and process-driven now. I am uncertain if this is a good or bad thing: good, because it is a more level playing field; bad, because it excludes the maverick!

Andrew introduced me to his colleague Michael Edgar, who was very different. He wasn't tall, but he was the quintessential Englishman. A devout Protestant and great supporter of the arts, and a thoroughly good man. Michael took me on as a registrar at the Middlesex Hospital, and subsequently appointed me as his consultant colleague there. My time at the Middlesex Hospital, with its formal rounds, and the iron hand of Sir Rodney Sweetnam (subsequently president of the Royal College of Surgeons), provided a first-class training, and a great introduction to the practice of surgery.

Of the many anecdotes given to us by Sir Rodney, I remember one in particular, which taught me that things are not always what one would expect in an interpersonal interaction. The first involved a patient with a condition called hallux valgus (a bunion of the big toe). This usually affects both feet. At this time, remedial surgeries were performed on one foot at a time, for obvious reasons. Sir Rodney didn't realise that his elderly patient suffered a marked lack of blood supply to her feet, I believe due to diabetes. In the process of performing the operation on one of her feet, the big toe ceased to have blood and subsequently had to be amputated. Sir Rodney said that usually in these circumstances, although the patients themselves are quite stoical about the outcome, they are persuaded by friends, colleagues and relatives to bring a claim against the surgeon. Indeed, he was expecting one at any moment.

As time passed, he saw the patient several times in clinic. On one of these occasions, the patient said to him, 'Well, Mr Sweetnam, I am afraid the last time you undertook surgery to my right foot, you had to amputate my big toe.'

Ah, here it comes, thought Sir Rodney.

'Although unfortunate, I must tell you that the operation was a great success,' the patient continued. 'I wonder if you could amputate my big toe on the other side?'

A similar episode occurred to me. As part of my practice in spinal surgery, I administer epidural and facet injections that provide pain relief to a large number of patients. One of the patients I saw in my clinic was the lawyer involved in determining the planning application for the new build of my hospital. She came to see me because she had intractable back pain, and after examining her, I felt it would be reasonable to proceed with an epidural.

It is my usual practice to train my trainees in injections, and I had a particularly enthusiastic trainee who took to the procedure quickly. In fact, when the patient's turn came, the trainee administered the injection before I had even entered the room. All seemed well initially, but when the patient returned to the ward, we received a call saying she was going blind.

We examined her and, sure enough, there were large sub-retinal haematomas (bleeding into the eye), and the consensus was that the injection had been given with such force that this had caused the bleeding. All involved, including my poor anaesthetist, were distressed by this, as was the hospital's medical director. We transferred the patient rapidly to Moorfields Hospital for the examination of her eyes and treatment of her retinal haematomas. I heard nothing for a year. Then, one day, the patient turned up in my clinic and I knew my time had come.

'Well, Mr Noordeen,' she said, 'you know, the last time you gave me injections I nearly went blind.'

I nodded gravely.

'However,' she continued, 'fortunately the staff at Moorfields were able, with the use of lasers, to get rid of the bleeds completely and totally restore my sight.'

I breathed a deep sigh of relief and congratulated her.

Then, rather than handing me a notice of her legal action, she told me she was so grateful for the injection – which had relieved her back pain – that she wondered if she could have another, as the pain was now beginning to return. We did give her a second injection, but this time I ensured it was administered by me, and I am delighted to say I haven't seen her since.

• • •

Ernie Kirwan was an Englishman, I believe of Irish origin, whom I had the privilege of meeting in my training, and from whom I learnt very different lessons. He was one of the most successful surgeons in Harley Street, and he performed two operations to perfection. The first was a hip replacement, and he did it well, usually in around forty minutes. The second was a discectomy and decompression, the most basic of spinal operations, for which he had a great success rate. As a consequence, he had a wonderful reputation. Any complex patients were referred to one of his colleagues (usually Andrew Ransford), on the grounds that they were far better qualified to look after them. The success rate with more complex patients was, understandably, significantly less.

One of the most memorable episodes during my apprenticeship as a registrar (currently grade ST2) to Ernie – or Mr Kirwan, as he was known to me then – was when a patient came to our clinic with severe back pain and sciatica (pain running down her leg), which had put her in a wheelchair. She was of Turkish origin and she was accompanied by all her family, who informed me that she had been in this state for six months. I arranged for her to have an MRI scan, and this revealed a large disc prolapse.

I showed her scans to Ernie, who simply asked, 'How long has she had this?'

'Six months,' I replied.

'Why hasn't she sought advice earlier?'

I shrugged my shoulders and repeated his questions to her family, who said they wanted her health to be treated conservatively and had tried alternative treatments until this point.

Ernie nodded sagely and said to me, 'Well, why don't you decompress her, remove the disc and try to alleviate her symptoms?'

I discussed this with her relatives, and they agreed to have the procedure done.

The patient was admitted a few days later, and imagine the joy of her family when she was out of bed and walking without pain, wandering around the wards. She went home a few days later – again, much to the joy of her family. I saw them in clinic after a few weeks: her symptoms were greatly improved, and she was feeling well.

Several months later, she was referred back to the clinic with a recurrence of her symptoms. Much to my dismay, I saw she was back in her wheelchair. I questioned her, asking whether she had any pain, and she said that she did not. What she did tell me, however, was that given the attention she had from her family, she felt she could not cope *without* being in the wheelchair, despite the fact that she wasn't in pain. To a large extent, she felt a wheelchair existence suited her.

An MRI scan confirmed there was no recurrence of her problem and Mr Kirwan discharged her, again nodding sagely. This provided an abject lesson to me: it is astonishing how quickly people can get used to certain behaviours that might lead to their benefit, then find it difficult to get out of the habit, even when the original problem has been solved.

The back pain clinics were held on a Friday afternoon, and were much dreaded by generations of registrars and junior registrars (doctors in training, on their way to specialist training). As the afternoon wore on, all those providing the service slid lower behind their consulting desk, weighed down by patient after patient with seemingly unending back pain, showing no sign of remission.

On one such occasion, a clinic that started around lunchtime went on quite late, and at six o'clock I sent for the last patient: an elderly woman who had attended the clinic for many years with a condition called ankylosing spondylitis. It was an inflammatory condition of the spine, which at that time had no possible cure, and the only available remedies were in the management of its complications, which included significant deformity of the spine. In this patient's case, she'd had no previous surgery but was nevertheless debilitated by her painful condition.

I recall asking the young nurse to go and fetch the last patient. She rushed back in a state of acute agitation, announcing that she had found the patient dead in her chair. I approached the formidable Sister Hunter, who ran the outpatient clinic in Bolsover Street, and we arranged for a set of screens to be placed around the patient, who was in a sitting position, already in a state of rigor mortis. The patient and her chair were then discreetly brought into the clinic, where she remained frozen in situ until the ambulance came and took her to University College Hospital. This was the first and last time I have ever encountered a patient who died while waiting to be seen!

The UK is characterised by the rule of law. Engendered by generation after generation of both lawmakers and lawgivers, it is a complex, dialectical system characterised by:

1. Thesis and antithesis.
2. The severe chastisement of both falsehood and corruption.
3. A certain rigidity in the way in which the law is applied.
4. Judgements that allow a degree of interpretation of the law and a latitude for clemency.

Mrs Thatcher once said that the British on the whole thought that people should receive what they deserve, but never what they want. This viewpoint has positive aspects, including the remarkable patience that the British show in the process of queueing, whether it be at a bank, at a post office, the bus stop or on a waiting list, awaiting their care on the National Health Service.

Patience can be taken to a remarkable extent. That it can be taken to the extent where a patient could die while waiting to be seen in clinic is, frankly, preposterous. Equally preposterous was the fact that none of the staff, and none of the other patients who were also waiting so patiently around her, noticed she had died.

CHAPTER SIX

Opioids Have Become the Religion of the Masses

Between the conception
And the creation
Between the emotion
And the response
Falls the shadow
For Thine is the Kingdom
'The Hollow Men' by T.S. Eliot

A darkness has descended upon the very practice of everyday medicine. To understand the nature of this malaise is to get to the root of every aspect of the contemporary medical universe.

When I did my general practice stint as a medical student, I was asked by my wise trainer in rural Oxford to make a note of the type of complaint that patients came in with. Only two-thirds were genuine medical complaints. A third of the patients came in simply to have a chat.

There has been a tremendous decline in church attendances, the priesthood and attendance at confession. In modern industrialised society, where, ironically, Karl Marx described religion as the 'opiate of the masses', opioids have indeed become the religion of the masses.

There has been an increased urge to classify just about every human condition. Every state of the human psyche, whether it be temporary or permanent, has a classification. Extreme happiness becomes euphoria and deep sadness, depression.

A friend of my mine once said that most American doctors work on the premise that every single American believes that for any condition, the remedy consists of either a pill or surgery. In other words, there is nothing a doctor cannot cure.

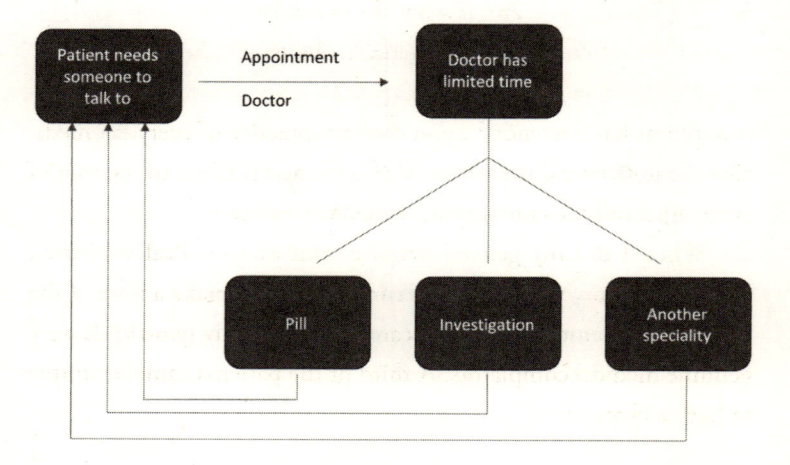

You can see that a GP consultation has been used as a means of social interaction, or at least a listening post. A vicious cycle has been set up, and the system perpetuates itself. The only way of getting anyone to listen is via consultation, either by making an appointment or, in the US, by means of payment. Increasingly, the amount of time that doctors have to listen, particularly to social issues, has become limited. All consultations have to be done in a certain time and are usually brought to an end by means of a pill or a referral for further treatment. This is a false economy. The cost in terms of both money and time is enormous. The social cost of sending a patient for ever more expensive investigations, or medications, or another referral, just to get them out of the consulting room, is huge. And then the exact same thing happens at the next consultation.

The classification of emotional states has become the norm, both by clinicians and by the media. As soon as most individuals reach their home, or indeed are en route, they are in front of their screen or their phones. The thing that they are becoming incapable of doing is thinking. There is an inability to meditate. There is a reluctance towards any form of introspection to even try to understand what it is that might be causing their emotional state, and dealing with it at a fundamental level. Most don't even know how to begin. It is easier to find this through a paradigm or an algorithm, allowing a quick fix of a problem.

Every emotional state has thus become classified. By classifying, this has medicalised it. By medicalising it, the responsibility or need for introversion and self-discipline has been removed, and the onus of treatment put on an outside source. The remedy for this could be a pill, or surgery, or cognitive behavioural or other form of therapy. At any rate, there is little emphasis on individual responsibility. It is therefore no wonder that consultation by an increasingly incapable medical community, due either to time constraints, algorithms, care pathways, or a lack of education in empathy, can be terminated with medication or indeed referral for some other form of therapy. Ultimately, the fundamental cause of this malady comes down to a belief that an emotional state can be medicalised into some form of disease.

The belief that any disease can be cured has now taken root. Whether the 'cure' consists of a pill, therapy, alcohol or drugs, this habitual use of medication becomes the norm, an addiction. This addiction leads to an increase in the volume of whatever drug or substance is used to toxic levels. This toxicity can lead to physical organ failure and death, and in this way, sometimes the remedy can be as devastating as the original symptoms.

What has been the approach to this vicious cycle? Further classification. Further medicalisation. The ability to access drugs in a 'safe' manner.

I was always impressed by the way in which Alcoholics Anonymous and Narcotics Anonymous function. Their approach to the issue is:

1. To promote recognition by each individual at every session that they have a problem.
2. To help improve the ability to interact at a social level, and enable others to help themselves at a human level.

I am astonished at the paucity of research on the effectiveness of these organisations, or at least any publicity regarding this. Still, it begs the question: if all this treats is the effect, what will be the treatment of the cause?

* * *

I grew up in a world in which there were no televisions, no mobile phones and no computers. Every day, my siblings and I returned home from school and engaged with our parents in some form of conversation, because there was literally nothing else to do. If we didn't want to do that, then the only alternative was to go out and play cricket with our cousins, or indeed stay late at school. School would start at

7 a.m. and finish at 1.30 p.m. Lunch would always be eaten together as a family, after which we would have an afternoon nap, followed by a whole host of 'supplementary tuition' and teachers, dinner, again with our parents, and then bedtime. We had to develop our art of conversation both with our parents and with our siblings.

This is in direct contradiction with what is happening at the moment. We have great difficulty as a family in preventing our children from watching TV, and the easiest thing to do is to come home after a hard working day and eat dinner in front of the television. (I, too, was guilty of doing this before my children arrived.) The television initially became a substitute for conversation and subsequently has become a substitute for thought, along with social media, video games, and other activities that take place from behind a screen.

Things have become far worse. I can hardly type and am almost dyslexic when it comes to sitting in front of a computer screen. There is nothing I dislike more than doing this. This again is in contradistinction to our children.

This shift towards dependence on technology is reflected in the hospital setting. Most communication is now 'paperless', whereas I still spend a great deal of time writing letters to friends and family, often to thank people for their hospitality or to express my condolences. I fear that my children will one day cease writing altogether. Certainly, in the hospital setting, writing is greatly discouraged and all requests and communications must be either by email or via filling in various forms on drop-down menus on a computer screen.

This has now become a general malaise in society. We live in a Facebook or Twitter culture and all of life can be conducted in front of a screen or virtually. Even among my colleagues who are interviewing patients, their primary focus is on the screen rather than on the patient. Social media is a tool for living a virtual life.

Anything that anyone wants to be known about themselves or others is posted on Facebook. Communication is a series of inane updates, all expressing a single proclamation rather than any depth of emotion. Many people now live in a totally virtual world. A soulless world. The value of anything is measured by the value of one's wealth (quantity), by one's productivity (the number of cases that one can do, or the number of patients one can see in a day), or one's popularity (the number of 'likes' generated on social media).

We have a target-driven society, whether one has to see a certain number of patients or bring in an income determined by 'session'. The motivation for conforming to the new norms, of course, is fear. The fear of losing one's job. The fear of attracting complaints. The fear of investigation. Work that is a means to an end in terms of doing something that is satisfying has been overturned by the means to the end. Work is done for work's sake and the driver is now the most basic instinct of fear.

In our screen-based, two-dimensional 'virtual society', we have lost the art of any form of face-to-face communication involving not only verbal interaction but also the ability to calibrate our intuitive resources (which requires the irreplaceable presence of human beings). That is the paradigm under which modern society works. Social relations are now driven by a near-total lack of meaningful communication, conversations being conducted either by email or telephone. Even when communication is face to face, what was said or the implications of what was said can only be established once it is confirmed in an email or text.

Earlier in my career, I was told by an astute manager that whichever manager I met, and whatever was said in any meeting, should be documented and put on the record. He cleverly indicated that some of the things on the record may or may not have been said, and if unchallenged, would nevertheless become part of the record. So now we have:

1. A lack of direct, face-to-face communication with any degree of meaning.
2. Communication that is stunted by a need to document what has been said, even to the extent of documenting the nuances.
3. An ingenuity and cunning introduced into any form of record in which 'spin' can be added to any conversation, which may have been conducted in a completely different spirit, and which may have had an entirely different meaning.

No wonder, then, that the average individual in distress, with their guard down and at their most vulnerable, who communicates their vulnerability, risks a communication that will be interpreted in a certain way and documented in a certain way. Furthermore, any form of communication now has to be classified. Every emotional state comes with an ICD (International Classification of Disease) classification attached.

We now have a society in which not only is the measure of an individual's worth literally a measurement of wealth, height, weight, postcode and birthdate, but also, any non-empirical communication – for example, that of emotion – needs to classified and analysed. A classification (algorithm) has been undertaken: often this is a mechanical process and may be conducted as part of a system using a whole series of drop-down boxes finely classifying a potential complaint. This produces a dangerous combination of:

1. The need to classify everything.
2. The need to have an algorithm for any form of remedy.

3. The understanding that once everything is classified, the remedy is easily identified and usually this involves a pill, therapy or referral.

Given that the whole process is driven by fear (in that one has to be productive), a GP, for example, may only have a ten-minute slot in which to hear a complex personal problem. The pressure is immense. No wonder then that the easiest option is to immediately categorise, classify and 'box' any conversation, and to follow this up with some form of prescription, whether it be a pill, therapy or referral. This is the current paradigm of care.

I know few clinicians who are able to say with any degree of equanimity that they are unable to do something, as they are terrified that their very competence may be thrown into doubt.

You can imagine that if one were to say to the vast majority of patients attending a back pain clinic that there is little that you, the doctor, can do for them, both the patient and the management might come to the conclusion that you were simply incompetent. We are drawing close to a situation where the whole of the medical establishment might have to come clean, particularly in terms of their management of pain, and admit that the available tools are limited, and may even cause harm. 'First, do no harm.'

It is not unusual for my colleagues and me, particularly those of us who work in tertiary referral centres, to refer patients to have numerous surgeries, each causing either the same or a greater degree of pain. The hardest task is to tell a patient that there is nothing further that can be done. The patients have such high expectations that one can identify clearly the origin of their pain, which is rarely the case, particularly in the context of repeat surgery. Even if the origin is clear and surgery is possible, it is often impossible to reduce the pain from a series of failed surgeries. It is unfortunately a case of a triumph of hope over experience.

It is difficult for a patient not to be dragged into this spiralling folly, and in many cases, doctors – and I am as guilty as anybody else – take on cases where there is little chance of successfully curing pain. To say that at least one tried may assuage one's own conscience, but again, 'First, do no harm'. It takes a brave surgeon indeed to admit his limitations.

This is a corporate culture that always existed outside of the NHS. The NHS was immune for precisely the reason that it was a 'sacred cow'. The drivers for healthcare in many developed countries are both financial, in terms of reward, and litigation, in terms of punishment. Indeed, we have a strange paradigm within the NHS where, however productive an individual is, everyone is paid precisely the same. There are, nevertheless, targets. What is missing in all of this is that indefinable but most important value: quality. The measurement of outcomes is of little value except as a means of measurement of complication and therefore cost. Patient experiences and a systematic review of patient experience – and most importantly, patient expectation – are required.

How does one measure quality? The measurement of quantity, of outcomes, does little apart from pay lip service. The quotation and systematic review of patient experiences, with all the nuances that help evoke the quality of the 'human touch', are required. Nevertheless, the problem is much more fundamental, with expectations that can rarely be met, either in the promptness and efficacy of treatment or in the outcomes.

Patient expectations are the elephant in the room. These are rarely verbalised but, when unmet, are a cause of deep unhappiness, disappointment, despair and sometimes litigation. However good an outcome is, if it fails to match expectation, it is of no value whatsoever. Any treatment must involve an explicit agreement that states both a clear understanding of expectation and likely (or unlikely) outcomes. This is the only sustainable means of delivering a service.

This is the very heart of the matter. Expectation and outcome. A contract. A contract based on a clear articulation of expectation with a clear articulation of outcome. What is present now is simply an articulation of outcome in terms of risks and benefits, with an expectation on the part of the clinician that the patient (or 'client') will behave as one does in a shop or a mall, where 'let the buyer beware'. I do not think that medicine, which works at a much more intimate and profound level, can or should operate in this way. It is important not only to explicitly state possible outcomes – or 'risks' – but also, as part of a contract, for there to be an explicit statement of expectation. Simply saying 'I wish to be better' is of no value. It is important as part of the process of consent to treatment to have expectation verbalised as explicitly as possible. This may require some form of interlocutor – perhaps a patient advocate. What is interesting is when I see non-English-speaking patients with an interlocutor or interpreter present. I am able to discern and ascertain much more of the patient's expectations, as the interlocutor in these circumstances is often able to verbalise them clearly. Nowhere in the modern consent form is there an articulation of expectation.

Is it too much to ask in the NHS setting, where the patient no longer belongs to an individual clinician but rather to the trust or hospital, that the only entity who is not in a consultation, the organisation (i.e., the hospital or trust), should be represented by a patient advocate?

Is it then too much to ask that time, space and the process of consent have patient expectation clearly articulated by the patient, guardian or advocate?

CHAPTER SEVEN

The Crowning Virus That Changed Everything

The word 'corona' means crown. The novel coronavirus SARS-CoV-2, which causes the disease named COVID-19, appeared in Wuhan province in China (where, incidentally, there is a germ warfare facility). The origins of this virus are uncertain, and of course there are several conspiracy theories. However, the first we knew about it was when China announced a lockdown of a number of cities for several weeks. Videos came through of new hospitals being built to accommodate the large number of cases, and this unprecedented move from China did alert us, or at least should have alerted us, to the extreme seriousness of this viral outbreak. To make matters worse, we had a leadership in the US that not only had denied climate change, but also denied that this particular virus was going to have any serious impact at all.

What do we know about this virus? Most flu viruses originate in China, where the viruses incubate and mutate in pigs and, given the close proximity between pigs and humans, are passed on by airborne droplets. The majority of us will have a mild viral flu-type illness with an increased temperature and a cough, which may be persistent, and we will then get over it. As to how long after this we will continue to shed the virus is uncertain.

Even if a vaccine or quick test were discovered today, the problem would be how to manufacture it to scale in the shortest time. For a vaccine, one would normally go to a vaccine manufacturer already making, say, the vaccine for the flu virus. That manufacturer will respond that they already have a thriving business, but:

1. They need to get new equipment, usually from China, which is in lockdown, and who is going to fund them and procure the equipment for them in the interim?
2. What is to happen to all those vulnerable people who may die of the flu because resources for making the flu vaccine have been diverted?

So the government will end up having to requisition financially or via those companies at enormous cost. Then the virus will mutate (in China first, as most flu viruses do) and we will need a different vaccine, as we do for flu every year. Testing is no different. You get the idea. The true incidence of the disease in the population is difficult to ascertain, particularly in underdeveloped countries, and the only valid parameter is the death rate and those already in the intensive care units.

What is certain is that the coronavirus has changed the world. The whole aviation industry has been scaled down to a large extent. Many workers in the hospitality industry and in aviation have been laid off. As I write, twelve million people signed up for social security in Canada three days ago, and it is very likely that twenty million people will have signed up for social security in the US. The markets have been negatively impacted. The point is, no one understands how to value assets and more in this new paradigm. The whole world economy is likely to be changed. It is impossible for me to be precise as to the effect on the world, but perhaps I can give some pointers as to how the practice of medicine will change.

There are patients who are not affected by the coronavirus – for example, those with heart attacks and strokes and cancer – that need to be treated, and while the coronavirus epidemic is at its peak it is likely that these patients will face unnecessary suffering and possible death. There will be a whole host of these patients who require treatment once the epidemic has been contained. How this is delivered remains an issue and there will need to be a new social contract as to how these patients are treated and how rationing (which will be inevitable in these circumstances) will be applied, because many of the industries that produce equipment and drugs for other conditions will have been repurposed for the treatment of COVID-19, resulting in a shortage of these items.

In England, the private sector was requisitioned for treating coronavirus cases, to the extent that one could not do anything other than urgent care in that sector, while the focus of the manufacturing industry was on building respirators. Again, this is something that cannot be switched on and off, and it will take a good year to return to their normal manufacturing habits.

Doctors and nursing staff are being increasingly focused on becoming carers for the intensive care crisis that is looming with respect to the management of coronavirus patients. Once the crisis abates, it will again take a while to reassign and retrain them for a return to normal practice, which will reach monumental proportions with the massive waiting lists there will be for treating other conditions, which may include certain cancer treatments. This will be repeated serially with each wave of the virus.

There are moments in a medical career where everything changes. This is one of those moments. The reality of modern medicine has been irrevocably transformed, and we do not have neither the time nor the tools to mourn our old lives, nor the tools to grieve.

It has been widely acknowledged that many junior doctors are facing burnout given the challenges of working extended hours under intense stress and with such high emotional stakes. Due to sheer unprecedented numbers, the resulting de-personalisation of the team that delivers care has swiftly accelerated the sense of being a cog in the corporate wheel. The attendant absence of structure also leaves doctors isolated from one another, threatening the all-important spirit of collegiality that ordinarily fuels morale.

It's difficult to convey palpable empathy or make a diagnosis via Zoom or Microsoft Teams – and next to impossible to read people's fears or intuit the unsaid.

Which begs the question: how does one grieve either individually or collectively on screen, so that we may come terms with our new reality?

I have already identified the way in which medicine can change. The precise nature of these changes will depend very much on how quickly the vaccine, or an anti-viral, can be developed to treat this, and whether the fundamental issue as to viral load makes a difference as to the severity of the outcome. It is easy to identify the various problems that will no doubt arise and that will change fundamentally not only how society, but how every single one of us lives and the way in which we as doctors practise medicine. I cannot precisely predict the form, although I have indicated some of the things that might be different.

Living in space and time one has to be someone, somewhere, at a particular time. What matters is to understand that within each of us is a life-giving and -saving essence that is unique to our particularity. We need to be in contact with this positive essence. The question is how to actualise this, to draw life from our source. A tree must always have contact with its root. A trusted and constant method, together with virtue, guarantees well-being. In a tree, the well-being of the trunk, through the flow of the sap, is an essential part of the trunk with its roots.

Part II

THE CRISIS

CHAPTER EIGHT

Alienation

Our dried voices, when
We whisper together
Are quiet and meaningless
As wind in dry grass
Or rats' feet over broken glass
In our dry cellar
'The Hollow Men' by T.S. Eliot

To be listened to. To be acknowledged. To be conversed with. Ultimately, to gain empathy. This is also to have shared ownership of a dialogue. In *Macbeth*, Shakespeare states, 'Life's but … a poor player / That struts and frets his hour upon the stage / And then is heard no more…' The point is that to live, one has to converse.

A problem shared is a problem halved. To get something off one's chest. There is no question that conversing and simply putting the issue or problem out there helps both the speaker and the listener gain insight into the issues. Understanding the nature of the problem goes a significant way towards determining a remedy, from the point of view of both the narrator and the listener.

Conversation, empathy and diagnosis have now been replaced by either an algorithm or an MDT (Multi-Disciplinary Team) meeting. In the distant past, every individual was his own priest and intimately involved in what was going to happen to him. He would search for the answers within himself and through himself, with the help of spiritual guidance given by tradition. Now, one's efforts to overcome the problems of everyday life are directed not by spiritual guides but by impersonal institutions. It doesn't have to be spiritual, but it does have to be personal. The result is not only a somatisation of emotion through illness, but also an inability to make an accurate diagnosis of one's ailments, their causes, and thus, an effective and permanent cure. There is a serious disconnection.

Life is moving, in 'virtual' channels, away from humanity and towards inhumanity. For what is more inhuman than to think we are communicating with our fellow human beings when all we are doing is exchanging digitalised computer images? There is no longer an interpersonal dialogue; instead, we have impersonal communication: we are led to believe that we can text or email an emotion, a state of being, a mode of consciousness, a human feeling. The truth is that it is much more complex.

All requests for medical tests must now be logged on a screen and online. There is a paperless consultation and a paperless request for investigations. Most of the time, rather than looking at a patient, a clinician or other professional will be looking at a screen. They will be typing their notes on a keyboard as they listen to – rather than look at – the patient, trying to assimilate abstract information instead of empathising with human emotion. Body language gives us so much information, but in a medical consultation it is so often ignored.

Everything today, ranging from a football match to a major world event, is subjected to commentators expressing opinions. Conversation has been abrogated to a screen or texting, or to Facebook, Instagram or Twitter. Thought and commentary has been handed over to commentators or people who are 'followed' on social media. Indeed, I am astonished as to how even children at a very early age are taught computer skills at the expense of language skills or the art of communication, or the ability to simply read an individual's face. An inability to understand or to read facial expressions gives an individual a form of autism, which is ultimately an inability to empathise. No wonder then, since once cannot read emotion in others, that one fails to understand the emotion in oneself. No wonder that, when there is an inability to understand or control one's own emotion, there is a somatisation – that is, the expression of psychological distress by the presence of physical symptoms – which is then treated as a physical illness.

An inability to deal with emotion is classified as a disease, and given an 'International Classification of Disease' classification. When something is classified as a disease, the remedy must be in the form of a tablet or injection. Thus we have the medicalisation of emotion – the medicalisation of what in the past would have been considered an ordinary part of daily life, a life full of ups and downs, emotional highs and lows.

What is taking over is a medical-industrial complex that creates bespoke medication, able to deal with emotion that is both uncontained and, at an individual level, unfathomable. It either suppresses this emotion or transforms it into some form of data susceptible to empirical analysis that can then be classified. Once classified, of course, it can be 'treated', often with some formulation of drug. When there is this possibility, there is then the necessity of manufacturing the drug, marketing the drug and selling the drug.

The algorithm works in favour of the medical-industrial complex. What has happened is disempowerment on an enormous scale of an individual's ability to deal with their own mental, and thus physical state, for our mental state is inextricably tied to our physical state. Hence, when one walks into a consultation room, there is a limitation on the time spent in the consultation. Within this time frame there is an algorithm that determines what the outcome of that consultation is likely to be – presumably some form of treatment or referral for treatment.

In order for this to occur, there has to be categorisation or a classification of the nature of the consultation. This is usually performed in front of a screen and involves what the patient says. Rarely does it involve what the patient has not said, has not been given the chance to say, does not have the capacity to say – to the very person whose job it is to help the patient understand their ailment as a prelude to healing it.

What someone *hasn't* said is usually as important as what *is* said. What is unsaid usually resides within the body: there is a body language, and not just facial expressions, that the doctor is no longer capable of reading. We are not trained to read anything other than empirical data. Reading the human being in depth no longer has meaning in the medical profession.

Communication involves both verbal and non-verbal interaction. The most difficult thing to fathom in modern society is non-verbal communication. This is because one simply doesn't have the capacity to do so. All algorithms are based on empirical truth, the truth of what can be measured. The proof of measurement lies in the ability to use a ruler or a scale, or other means of measurement. What is incapable of measurement, therefore, is classified as being unreal.

All emotions, be they anger or hate or love, happiness or sadness, would be ultimately unmeasurable, and must by their definition be empirically unreal.

This one-sided view of reality as being empirical has tremendous consequences that can be devastating to the individual, in that, unfortunately, any form of empirical approach to something that is fundamentally unmeasurable is doomed to failure. This whole process is then exacerbated by the culture of entitlement.

An empirical reality means a reality that can only be measured via the senses, i.e. smell, taste, hearing, touch and sight. Since most emotion cannot be measured, this empirical approach to the unmeasurable will fail. By its nature, entitlement is a sentiment, an emotion. How can one measure what it is that an individual wants or is entitled to?

In the nanny state, where the state looks after our pension, our health, our education, there is an expectation of entitlement. This entitlement includes that every condition – every somatisation – should have a remedy and must be looked after.

Ultimately, this is alienation. An alienation from the ability to understand one's own emotional or physical state, together with the dangerous consequences of the abrogation of its understanding, its analysis and its treatment to an algorithm, or to an empirical phenomenon, which cannot by definition approach or possibly remedy something that is not within its reach. Add entitlement to alienation. There then comes a deep sense of loss and of grief. The result is a loss of ownership of both the means and the end of any endeavour.

A loss of ownership of conversation, a loss of ownership of dialogue, a loss of ownership of process, a loss of ownership of a potential solution or remedy. A loss of the ability to empower oneself. A loss of a sense of achievement in solving a problem by oneself. An absence of effort.

Whole industries have grown up around each of these failures. Social media has taken ownership of conversation – at the end of the day, someone is benefiting from every digitalised exchange, and this is very much a commercial activity. Industry has taken ownership of the process of classification of any form of disease, including somatised disease.

Industry has also taken ownership of the algorithm that now exists for the treatment of disease. Commerce has taken ownership of any remedy that may be available, whether it be cognitive behavioural therapy or a drug that may be used to alter or control moods. This is not to say that an antibiotic used judiciously is not of great value. It is simply to say that the whole process of being commercialised has meant the loss of ownership to the individual, hence alienation.

When I was a trainee, a multi-disciplinary meeting to discuss disease and remedy involved taking a history – that is, to systematically obtain a chronology and context from a patient. The patient was then seen and examined by all the clinicians involved. The diagnosis and potential treatment options often involved the patient. In a modern multi-disciplinary meeting, the one person who is not in the room is the patient. Alienation. Disconnection from reality. A life in a virtual world.

An abrogation of personal responsibility is inevitably a loss of ownership. A loss of responsibility, or to give away one's responsibility over one's thoughts and actions, is a loss of ownership of one's life.

* * *

How, then, shall beauty save the world? Darkness occurs in a system where the means becomes the end. Most students go into medicine with the ultimate aim of delivering care. What they will end up with, if they do not take heed, is practising medicine for the sake of practising medicine. The same problem – confusing the means for the end – can happen to any human process, including those processes that take place within religious institutions.

Religion has always been a means of establishing a portal between faith and a divinity; the root of the word shows this: 're-ligare' is to re-tie the bond between earth and heaven, humanity and divinity. But religion has also succumbed, in the modern world, to the degeneration that has taken over so many other processes. Instead of giving us illuminating truths, it has become a darksome force, a means that has become an end; religion for the sake of religion, instead of for the sake of God and humanity. Religion is now used as a tool to alienate the other while gratifying the self; to create divisions instead of building upon affinities. An ideology has grown around it that makes religion itself something that ends up violating the heart of faith, disfiguring the beauty of divinity, and undermining the meaning of humanity.

In my early youth in Sri Lanka, a predominantly Buddhist country, there was absolutely no doubt in my mind, and in the mind of all my Buddhist friends, that Buddhism was a religion comparable to my own, Islam, and to Hinduism and Christianity – the four main religions represented in Sri Lanka. None of us doubted for a second that we all believed in the same 'God', even if that ultimate Reality assumed different names, and was worshipped and meditated upon in different ways. We knew, instinctively, that what really mattered in the eyes of that ultimate Reality was not the name we called It, but how we translated our belief into virtue: how well our belief in that Reality expressed itself in our conduct as beauty. We seemed to be following different religions, but we all knew, in our heart of hearts, that we were striving for exactly the same goals; we were climbing the same mountain, but by different paths. This was best illustrated by all the faiths ascending the Sri Lankan mountain called Adam's Peak. At sunrise, the shadow of this magical mountain precedes it towards the sun. The Christians and Muslims believe it to be the footprint of Adam. The Buddhists, the Buddha. The Hindus, Vishnu.

Even if Buddhists officially rejected the idea of a Creator-God, we knew that their striving for the state of enlightenment was identical to our striving for salvation: both kinds of striving are motivated by the self-same state of consciousness, a state of absolute contentment with the deepest nature of things. And it was through the texture of our human interaction, the weaving of our real – not virtual – communication, our emotional and psychological state of 'entanglement' (to borrow a phrase from modern physics), that we understood how the oneness of our humanity, reflecting the oneness of Reality, so effortlessly (and gloriously) transcended the diversity of our religious beliefs. The unity of our faith and of the Divinity was 'proved' for us by the living, pulsating heart of our humanity.

But, alas, in our times, the heart of our humanity has become subject to a kind of spiritual sclerosis. Consequently, religion is no longer a heartfelt reality, but a fabricated ideology, a means not to any higher purpose, but a tool wielded only for the sake of self-aggrandisement, 'my' religion as opposed to 'yours'. In any process where the means becomes the end, a darkness will arise. This darkness can only be remedied by the light of beauty, by virgin nature, which is none other than the human being; and the quintessence of the human being, in turn, is the heart. The heart needs to be in a state to recognise this beauty, as beauty is in the eye of the beholder.

CHAPTER NINE

Culture of Care or Command and Control?

I learned that, most appropriately, the International Society for Suppression of Savage Customs had entrusted [Kurtz] with the making of a report, for its future guidance [...] it was a beautiful piece of writing. The opening paragraph, however, in the light of later information, strikes me now as ominous. He began with the argument that we whites, from the point of development we had arrived at, 'must necessarily appear to them (savages) in the nature of supernatural beings—we approach them with the might as of a deity' [...] This was the unbounded power of eloquence—of words—of burning noble words. There were no practical hints to interrupt the magic current of phrases, unless a kind of note at the foot of the last page, scrawled evidently much later, in an unsteady hand, may be regarded as the exposition of a method. It was very simple, and at the end of that moving appeal to every altruistic sentiment it blazed at you, luminous and terrifying, like a flash of lightning in a serene sky: 'Exterminate all the brutes!"

Heart of Darkness by Joseph Conrad

A darkness has descended into the National Health Service – in fact, into all healthcare systems. Much of the pre-NHS system consisted of charitably established or supported hospitals. Autonomy was given to the doctors and nurses to allocate resources to individuals' care. Care was locally based and locally responsive. Patients knew the matrons and consultants who were responsible for delivery of care, but resource reallocations were available where required – for example, if there was a cholera outbreak. This was in an environment of severe need with finite resources.

The term 'command and control' means that whoever is appointed to manage a service manages by ensuring compliance. It is also the means by which compliance is achieved. Methods include:

1. A culture of fear: if one is not compliant, one may be investigated, reprimanded, lose one's job, or at least go through some process of intimidation with the resulting insinuation being that one has done something wrong, something terrible.
2. Coercion: whether it be via some form of constructive dismissal or by more subtle means of bullying.
3. A power structure: establishing a hierarchy ensures that a hierarchical chain of command is followed – rather like the army, in that not to follow would involve some form of sanction.
4. Appointing compliant individuals to posts: individuals that would not challenge any precept, command or directive that comes from above.

How is this achieved?

1. First, one writes out a series of policies – for example, the GMC 'Good Medical Practice' – that can be used to get rid of an outlier,

even one who engages in good medical practice, on the grounds that one has failed to adhere to the small print, or at least where some parts can be used against an outlier.

2. By the use of various box-ticking exercises, where a whole series of actions needs to be checked. If this is not completed, then appropriate actions and sanctions are made. In this way, even laudable exercises, like the WHO Surgical Safety Checklist, can in turn – if a box is left unticked, for whatever reason – be used as a sanction or as a weapon. The WHO checklist is a series of questions that need to be answered before undertaking any procedure, with the aim of ensuring use of the correct equipment and procedure, and – most importantly – that the physical safety of the patient has been considered. To achieve higher compliance rates with the WHO checklist, managers should arrange appropriate mandatory training courses for workers, explaining and emphasising the importance of these checklists to patient care. Instead, consultants are threatened with public naming and shaming for low rates of compliance.

3. By doing a root cause analysis, looking at any occurrence and making it into a serious incident, or examining some form of activity for which the person undertaking the root cause analysis is both judge and jury.

4. Investigation for something as simple as being late for a clinic, to show that one is somehow defrauding the National Health Service. This lateness may well reflect legitimate NHS activities. For example, there has been a move in hospitals to conduct Multi-Disciplinary Team meetings to improve patient care. The creation of these meetings often leads to clinicians arriving late to clinics. Thus, lateness to clinics can be used as a reason to initiate an investigation, when in fact the lateness stems from an effort to improve patient care.

5. Appointing compliant individuals, perhaps individuals who may be too junior to understand the process and who are good at carrying out instructions, rather than those who have the ability to discern between a genuine and valuable request and one that is made either vindictively or aggressively as a means of expanding another's area of control.
6. Setting 'targets', which in some cases may be arbitrary and often unachievable, so that not achieving a target may in itself be deemed a punishable offence. Or indeed, if one does achieve it, one would do so at the expense of cutting corners and therefore exposing an individual or patient to some form of danger, which in itself could be punished in due course. An example of this would be the WHO checklist or the morning 'team brief' (part of the WHO checklist). These are time-consuming but laudable processes. However, if one is given a target of doing a certain number of cases or seeing a certain number of patients within a certain period of time, then one might necessarily exclude one or other of these processes. In doing so, one is open to direct action for having failed to carry out a certain process, for which one could suffer some form of punishment.
7. Divide and rule. Divisions can be engendered at several levels, such as the division between junior doctors and senior doctors. Sadly, it doesn't require managers to make this division. The junior doctors themselves organise and run this, and I am not arguing about the value of their cause or their aims. What I am saying is that this creates a division that can be and is exploited. Divisions can also be between departments. In any organisation in which resources are finite, you will find inevitable divisions, but again one must be acutely aware that they can be used as a means of command and control, as a means of compliance.

Divisions between individuals who may simply not get on, for whatever reason, can also be exploited, and the fallout from this becomes a spectacle, a distraction that allows interested individuals or organisations to carry out their ends while the saga is played out elsewhere. I don't know whether management is taught how to do this, but I am sure this type of disruption must have some sort of process to it!

8. Another way of ensuring compliance is by getting rid of a high-profile individual. This is a classic way of ensuring compliance. The reasoning behind this is to instil the fear that if it is possible to get rid of a well-known individual, then it could happen to anyone.

• • •

When I first started my career in medicine at Great Ormond Street twenty-two years ago, I had the good fortune of having an outstanding manager. I had taken over a service with a three-year waiting list for which no planning had been undertaken before I started my first day. We soon discovered that instruments (and there were over one hundred components required) had not been ordered and would not be available for several months. Having brought the first patient into the hospital for surgery, we simply had no means to operate on them. This was a disaster, both from the patient's point of view and from mine. What had been a three-year waiting list then became a three-year-and-three-month waiting list while we waited for the equipment required to operate on the patient. We reduced this where possible by borrowing equipment from the Middlesex Hospital and were able to operate on at least some of the patients on the waiting list, but not all. When the equipment turned up three months later, things finally got underway. In the interim, rather than twiddling my thumbs I began a series of dialogues with my immediate service manager, whose whole life had been fast-tracked as a management trainee at Great Ormond Street. In other words, he was a fast-tracked career manager, a new breed that was then coming into the National Health Service.

We made a plan. The first thing he told me, to my utter astonishment, was this:

'What you have got to realise, Mr Noordeen, is that we go on courses on how to deal with difficult doctors. We are taught that if we are in the process of implementing a directive and we have a doctor who is "uncooperative", we keep repeating the directive until the doctor potentially gets angry. If he were to even raise his voice a little, we would tell him that he was shouting. At this point you usually would shout. We would tell him that he was angry. At this point he really would become angry. At this point we would suggest that he went on an anger-management course, and that would either make him compliant or go completely over the top, at which point he would indeed be sent to an anger-management course. Our objective would be achieved.'

He paused, as I assimilated this unexpected information, my eyes wide.

'The best advice I can give you is that you must never say no. You must always say that you will think about it. When you go away, you must send us a memorandum documenting our conversation. You must then explain to us that you would be able to comply if other aspects of your service were to be resourced properly, enabling you to carry out this particular directive. You then give us a choice, which is either to resource you or not to be able to enforce your compliance. This is much more constructive because it then empowers me to go to my immediate superiors to get you the resources that you require. In that way, we both win.'

From that moment onwards, I ensured that any conversation I had with a manager was properly documented and sent to the manager thereafter. I never said 'no', I always said 'I'll think about it', and then told them under what circumstances I would be able to comply.

One concrete example of this was when, in my clinic, I needed to get through the large number of patients I was seeing (approximately twenty each morning). These were often new referrals. Fortunately, when I started, all requests, including blood requests, X-ray requests and attendance at the next clinic, were handwritten. All the X-rays came on hard X-ray sheets, which could be put up on a screen and looked at literally the moment the patient walked in. This was a very efficient process. We then moved to a paperless form of requests, with digitised X-rays, at Great Ormond Street. Again, all laudable in principle, but since I was at that time completely computer illiterate, it would have doubled the time necessary to see each patient. When the manager came to see me about this, I explained patiently what effect it would have on my service. I offered to either see half the number of patients that I would normally see, or to have a healthcare assistant to help me in the clinic, performing all my requests and freeing me up to concentrate on my clinical work. I got my healthcare assistant. The service went from strength to strength.

The other thing I did was to examine the reimbursement the hospital received for complex spinal operations, such as to treat scoliosis. The staff member of the billing department was a recent school leaver and really didn't know. Therefore, I asked her to tell me roughly what she thought the hospital might be paid. She asked me for the code for the procedure, which didn't exist (again, this was twenty-two years ago). She then suggested a code that she had for an operation on another part of the body (the foot), and came up with £2,000.

I promptly left the billing department and went and wrote up a care pathway, documenting the patient experience from the moment they walked into the hospital until the moment they walked out. Every consultation, including being seen by the junior doctors and clerking (history, examination, X-rays, investigations, blood tests), the cost of theatre time for every nurse present in theatre, the cost of the swabs, the cost of the various units of blood and fluids that were given during the procedure, the cost of the implants, and the cost of the care post-operatively, including being seen by the nurses, occupational therapists, physiotherapists, etc. My detailed analysis produced a figure of approximately £9,000. In that way, I worked out that we were losing out on approximately £7,000 per patient.

I went to see the then chief executive (an outstanding clinician and manager, Jane Collins), who quickly understood the implications of my care pathway. She rang the Department of Health, and to her amazement they had absolutely no idea what a spinal operation cost. We set up an inquiry to formally cost out spinal operations, which the Department of Health said they would be delighted to fund, and also pay a set rate that was found by any commission that we set up. We eventually determined that we should be paid £11,000 per case. Anything in excess of what was being used would go into the funds for the purchase of equipment, paying for extra trainees and funding research. What a wonderful model of decentralisation of a command and control structure, to the benefit of all concerned.

* * *

I believe that every single doctor should be taught to hold and manage his own budget. We have to do it at home for our personal finances; there is no reason why we can't do it for our practice.

In any paradigm that involves people being paid the same, however hard or however little they work, power or position eventually becomes currency. Your influence or power within the system is dependent not on how hard you work or how much money you bring in, but on your position within the structure. This is precisely what a communist state is. Power is the currency, rather than money. The NHS is a state within a state. It has its own rules and 'government', and is the largest employer in this country, whose numbers pretty much make it almost the size of a small state. It is a state in which everybody within certain bands is paid the same, and which carries with it a hierarchy akin to any apparatchik organisation that can be imagined.

The classic architect of the whole process of command and control within a bureaucracy is, of course, Stalin. His behaviour and the way in which he achieved compliance and control have been documented in many books and films. This message has not been lost on the NHS, who in fact use many of the techniques he practised, but of course they are articulated in terms that disguise the command and control ideology behind the mask of modern and postmodern political correctness. This is in the context of the NHS being a state within a state. The NHS, by statute, has its own set of rules, which at times are almost distinct to common law. A claim for unfair dismissal, for example, is successful, and has a payment that is capped, unlike other employments. Each trust has powers that would be a matter of concern in any other walk of life. Medical directors have powers that allow unprecedented latitude, without accountability, and make command and control possible.

• • •

I believe it would be an extremely good idea if clinicians were made aware of these techniques. I have publicly stated that it would be wonderful if all clinicians could go on a course called 'Managing the Managers'. I think the model that needs to be addressed is, of course, Stalin's model, and that will form the basis of an effective manual to deal with the inherent problems here.

In hindsight, the technique utilised by Stalin is predictable. When Stalin joined the communist party, he was pretty much a non-entity. There were several high-profile individuals, in terms of physical appearance, ability and intellect. He counted on two things:

1. The internal rivalry between these individuals.
2. Their arrogance.

Stalin was able to effectively remove them one by one, until he was the only one left. When Trotsky was removed from Stalin's path, hardly anyone opposed him.

This is often the template tacitly used by doctors who have gone into management, as they feel this would be a better career pathway than pursuing their profession on the basis of their ability as a doctor. There is an implicit recognition that it is not healing but succeeding that matters: care and compassion must be sacrificed to the idols of command and control.

What is the 'culture of care'? A culture of care is ultimately an enlightened self-interest. The currency becomes fulfilment, of doing a good job and being paid well for doing it. It is job satisfaction, or at least satisfaction by delivering good-quality care. This currency of satisfaction cannot be bought or replaced by money. This is true of every individual, and again, this is a non-empirical science. It is difficult to measure job satisfaction. The point about targets is that they are easily measurable. Satisfaction is not.

* * *

I believe the way to save the NHS from the poisonous ideology of command and control is through the antidote of care and compassion, practised not as if it were some new management initiative, but as a personal imperative. Healing should be the focus. Job satisfaction is just the tip of the iceberg. What is given to us, in depth, is an even more priceless commodity: total contentment and inner peace. We come closer to being true 'medicine men', in the sense understood so well in the Native American tradition, and indeed in all the traditional shamanistic societies. The medicine man was responsible for healing not just the body, but also the ailments of the soul, what we call today 'mental health issues'; and if he was not himself 'healthy', 'whole' and 'holy', how could he be expected to heal others?

The medicine man finds his equivalent in the Muslim world as the 'hakim', which means 'wise man' as well as physician. The true medicine man, the hakim, the healer, knows that it is only through his vision of the beauty of reality that he can become whole and content and receive inner peace. This vision of beauty has nothing to do with our empirical sight. Only the 'eye of the heart' can see this transcendent beauty.

Frithjof Schuon, a metaphysician, artist and poet who died in 1998 at the age of ninety, recounts the following words spoken to him by Black Elk, a medicine man of the Oglala Sioux:

I am blind and I do not see the things of this world; but when the Light comes from On High, it illuminates my heart and I can see, because the Eye of the heart (Chante Ishta) sees all things. The heart is the sanctuary at the center of which is a small space where the Great Spirit (Wakan Tanka) lives, and this is the Eye of the Great Spirit by which He sees everything, and with which we see Him. When the heart is impure, the Great Spirit cannot be seen, and if you should die in this ignorance, your soul will not be able to return at once to the Great

Spirit, but will have to be purified by wanderings across the universe. To know the Center of the Heart where the Great Spirit dwells, you must be pure and good and live according to the way that the Great Spirit has taught us. The man who is pure in this way, contains the Universe in the Pocket of his Heart (Chante Ognaka).

***The Eye of the Heart* by Frithjof Schuon**

CHAPTER TEN

The Big Society

Re-establishing Care over Control

Anything approaching the change that came over his features I have never seen before and hope never to see again. Oh, I wasn't touched. I was fascinated. It was as though a veil had been rent. I saw on that ivory face the expression of sombre pride, of ruthless power, of craven terror—of an intense and hopeless despair. Did he live his life again in every detail of desire, temptation, and surrender during the supreme moment of complete knowledge? He cried in a whisper at some image, at some vision—he cried out twice, a cry that was no more than a breath—

'The horror! The horror!'

Heart of Darkness by **Joseph Conrad**

The politician Jesse Norman wrote a wonderful book called *The Big Society*. The book had simple ideals: every single individual should belong. They should belong to their society, their organisation, their community. It was all about being inclusive. To me, this is the antithesis of the culture of command and control. Put simply, it's how John Lewis runs their organisation. It is a partnership that involves everyone in the organisation, all of whom have ownership of the organisation. It is both a partnership and a cooperative.

At one time there was an idea that this 'big society' should be rolled out even to global organisations like the NHS. What it would have meant was that everyone in any trust or any GP practice (any employee, including the catering department, the cleaners, the healthcare assistants, the nurses, the doctors, the managers and so on) would have ownership and be stakeholders in the organisation. This would ensure that there was no command and control. This idea had short shrift, both within the Conservative party and within other organisations in government, particularly the NHS. That is a great pity. My thesis about the way in which we can restore the culture of care is based on a reversal of command and control, and the re-establishment of a culture of care by means of inclusivity and shared ownership.

Much is made of the words 'development' and 'progress' in the medical world. Development effectively means moving away from basic principles, and although it is necessary to move a certain distance from the principles in order to make applications of them, it is of vital importance to remain near enough for them to be fully effective. Development must never go beyond a certain point. How shall we presume not to live in fear of increasing our distance from the principles to the point where development becomes degeneration? What is proudly spoken of as development is, in many cases, very much a degeneration. The word 'progress' is often synonymously used with the word 'development'.

* * *

So what is the remedy? What is required is a renewal, or restoration, of the principles of care. The remedy is to recollect certain aspects of our established practice and to use this as a protective shell for the whole practice of medicine itself, for the delivery of care. We need to be consistently reminded of the dignity and responsibility incumbent on every practitioner, and they should be equipped regularly with these basic principles. To 'do no harm' would be a good start. To this effect, it is also important that the environment – the ambience in which we work – reflects that recollection. The outward acts upon the inward and there is no harm in even including a degree of formality to reflect a sense of propriety and dignity. Dignity in dress sense, dignity in action and dignity in the delivery of care.

It involves a reversal – in fact, a whole dismantling – of the tools of command and control. This has to happen from the top down, as follows:

1. A reversal of the artificial split between provider and commissioners.
2. Within organisations in the NHS (trusts), an end of the division between managers and clinicians, with common ownership of processes.
3. The setting up of care pathways to clearly establish process and to develop standardisation of care by means of care pathways that can be costed. Within care pathways there is plenty of opportunity for both diversity and innovation. As well as new drugs, new techniques and new instruments, innovation can also involve the way in which we work. Common ownership of the care pathway between all clinicians involved, including all levels of trainees, consultants, and so on, is vital. This does not exclude a hierarchy, but requires a hierarchy based on responsibility and inclusivity: firms within departments.
4. Devolving budgets to the different units within the organisation, and allocating responsibility over budgets. This includes train-

ing in the basics of budgeting and accountancy, which will help the individual not only at the level of the unit but also at a personal level.

5. A clear articulation of patient expectation must be documented. This goes hand in hand with the huge initiative on outcomes that is being carried out. A process of consent should include both expectation and outcomes, as well as a list of potential complications.
6. A return to an apprenticeship that is fundamentally training based, of which training in management and all the responsibilities of management, including budgets, are integral parts.
7. An education that is didactic and clinically orientated from the outset. This is not simply a series of lectures, but a teaching that is both unitary and integral.
8. A process by which every patient takes ownership of their pathway and thus of their disease.
9. Most important of all, a process of accountability, where all parties – patient, doctor and manager – are accountable for the pathway and its delivery.

In the last chapter, I referred briefly to the WHO checklist. This safety procedure was set up to ensure that a didactic process is followed prior to surgery, as follows:

a. That the patient has been properly prepared for the surgery.
b. That full consent is obtained prior to surgery.
c. That the appropriate site of surgery, X-rays and scans etc. are all available for the surgery.
d. That the surgery that was consented for is carried out.
e. That any equipment issues arising during surgery or untoward events are clearly documented, specified, and also action taken

to ensure that similar problems will not happen again, or can be minimised in the future.

f. After the operation, a sign-out procedure is carried out where the whole operation and its aftermath are reviewed and summarised.

The WHO checklist was established to minimise the avoidable errors that can arise during either the preparation for surgery or thereafter. I believe it is an extremely valuable tool.

How is it possible to reverse the split between providers and commissioners? This artificial division is a recent initiative. I think what is required, in a total and transparent manner, is:

1. A clear understanding of the resources available, fundamentally the budget.
2. To understand the cost of each and every service being provided.
3. A utilitarian decision supported by sufficient safeguards, including patients' organisations, the National Institute of Clinical Excellence, etc.
4. Within a speciality, a single process to prioritise aspects of care.

Ultimately, we should try to deliver the greatest good to the greatest number. Some decisions are exceedingly complicated. In a theoretical world where half the population are malnourished and the other half obese, would it be justifiable to offer, free at the point of delivery, surgery for obesity? Is it reasonable for the removal of tattoos to be available on the National Health Service? Some decisions seem obvious, but others are far more complex. Should gender reassignment be available on the National Health Service? These are value judgements that need to be taken individually and at a national level, but nevertheless, these are questions that should be made explicit and not become some form of political football.

* * *

It is easy to document and follow a template to track patient care. This has already been achieved in many specialities and is imperative both for the organisation to understand the resources required and the cost of these resources, and to empower the patient to understand the pathway and ensure they take ownership of their pathway. This has been made much easier by the use of iPads and various forms of social media in that it is no longer necessary, for example, to repeatedly come to hospital for physiotherapy when the patient is able to have their exercises supervised through the media at home. This is not difficult to achieve.

Once care pathways are established, it is a small step to cost and devolve them both at an individual level and to the different units and departments within hospitals. This is not meant as a competition, but as an explanation. It is important that every clinician understands what the delivery of their service costs, and what is being charged for their service. It is to take responsibility both at a personal level and at a collective level. It is ultimately the empowerment of the individual clinician. It is equally important that every patient knows the service they are getting and what their service costs. This transparency is critical to understand not only the cost of things but also the value of things. Nothing concentrates the mind as much as cost. Once cost has been established, it is a small step to establish value.

More than anything that has been articulated thus far, the whole aspect of patient expectation has been neglected. Outcomes have been studied ad nauseam. There have been randomised controlled studies, multi-variant analyses, case studies and systematic reviews, all to understand what the outcomes are and to justify whether a procedure should be carried out or not. This decision is being made in terms of cost, or indeed whether a particular procedure is better than doing nothing. The jury is still out as to whether the outcome for surgery for lower back pain is of any value or not. Billions of pounds are being spent on the treatment of chronic lower back pain, and it is rather strange that we are unsure as to whether it is of any significant benefit. I am sure if prioritisation was on an open and transparent basis that was at least utilitarian, many of these resources would be deployed elsewhere, or at least where they were most effective.

Nevertheless, the whole issue of patient expectation has never been addressed. It is crucial that we start a systematic study of what patient expectations involve. This is the best and most consistent way of giving patients ownership of their own pathway. Outcomes can only be contextualised in terms of expectation. Outcomes by themselves are simply a numerator without any form of denominator.

A systematic review of patient expectation in elective (as opposed to emergency) surgery should be undertaken. There needs to be some means of allowing every single patient to articulate their expectation of a procedure or consultation. There also then needs to be a clear contract as to what extent these expectations may or may not be met. I am astonished that it is possible to practise medicine in this day and age without explicit statements to this effect. Everything else is explicit. In the past, both expectation and outcomes were implicit. Now there is an imbalance in that we clearly understand outcomes to a large extent, but we don't at all understand expectations.

It is imperative, therefore, that training returns to being an apprenticeship as part of management, both at an individual level and at the level of the collective. During the apprenticeship, there should also be the ability to be trained in measuring both expectations and outcomes. Additionally, accounting and finance should become an integral part of any medical training, and should be maintained throughout. I am sure it would do no end of good at an individual level and at a collective level for the organisation, and for the NHS.

* * *

Medical education needs to take account of this idea of collective responsibility. Not only should it return to the basics of history and examination, but cost, value and expectation should become an integral part of all medical training. Already there are plenty of courses and processes that are able to measure and present accounting, finance and management to a student, trainee or practitioner, but nevertheless, this needs to be applied. What is lacking is a clear exposition and process of articulating expectation, and the ability to have some form of formal contract, matching expectation and the variety of possible outcomes.

All this needs to be inculcated and established in medical education from the outset. Personal teaching – face to face, one to one, with ongoing interaction – should become an integral part of medical education, and should be maintained throughout the process of apprenticeship.

Once there is a clear pathway for the caregiver, there should be a clear pathway for the patient. The aim is that the patient takes control not only of their pathway but also of their disease and its treatment. I think once patients understand that they have a clearly stated pathway, the treatment of their disease then becomes a lot easier to plan at all potential outcomes.

Every stakeholder in the organisation, including the patient, becomes an integral part of the care pathway. This involves every stakeholder taking responsibility and also being held accountable. This could mean something as simple as a failure on the part of a patient to attend a clinic, or failure of a unit or individual to administer care in a timely fashion. Either way, it is imperative that there is voluntary accountability at every step of the pathway.

In our quest to resolve some of the most pressing issues within medical practice, we must not be lulled into a false sense of security, thinking our efforts alone are sufficient reason to accept the lack of change that we see from day to day. It is important not to procrastinate and to make every single moment, every single day, count in terms of the fulfilment of our resolve. The best exposition of this is in the film *Groundhog Day*, which on the surface is about a tomorrow that never comes, but its deeper message is about making every tomorrow today – the one and only day. We will explore this deeper message within the next chapter.

CHAPTER ELEVEN

Groundhog Day

Every night I resolve: tomorrow,
I will abandon this passion.
But each time tomorrow arrives,
I turn today into another tomorrow again.
Badreddin Helali (a renowned Persian poet, d. 1529)

Everyone who goes into medicine will at some point experience their Groundhog Day. We seem doomed to repeat mistakes again and again, and each day seems like the next. How do we stop ourselves becoming a hamster on a wheel, and move forwards? More importantly, how can we engage with our day in order to change our tomorrow? How can we engage with our patients and colleagues, in order to change their tomorrows? On the level of an individual patient, there is empathy, where the other is 'none other than I'. What about the collective? What about our situation in that collective?

The 1993 film *Groundhog Day*, directed by Harold Ramis and starring Bill Murray, sends us the opposite message to the procrastination of which Helali complains. Instead, it tells us to make every single day the fulfilment of your resolution. The film is comic on the surface, and spiritual in depth, quite independently of the intentions of the scriptwriters – and therein lies its extraordinary power to move us.

On the surface, the film is about a tomorrow that never comes, but in depth, one sees it is about making every tomorrow today, the one and only day, thus inverting the message of the lines from Helali, and being truly, as the Sufis say, 'Son of the Moment'.

For Phil, the protagonist played by Murray, every 'tomorrow' is always Groundhog Day, the second of February. He never gets to the third day of February. At the end of each day, he sleeps, but always wakes up to the same day, Groundhog Day. But this occurs only for him; everyone else is acting as if it were Groundhog Day for the first time, as for them, it is. Phil alone has a repeated *déjà vu*, but he also has the freedom to change his behaviour as each day arrives. Because of his foreknowledge of what is going to happen, he also has the power to change those events... within limits.

The inability to escape from Groundhog Day at first gives rise to feelings of insanity, then recklessness, then indulging his lower appetites (for whatever be the actions today, they have no consequences for a tomorrow that never comes), then despair and attempted suicides. Still nothing stops tomorrow from being today, Groundhog Day, until at last the cycle is broken by his attainment of liberation through contentment in his ceaseless but now spontaneous effort at being the ideal image projected by his beloved.

If we have 'ears to hear', we can be, here and now, that which we desire. It just depends on what we desire, how deeply we care for it, and how much effort we are willing to expend in order to prove it. It is to become what we desire.

One of *Groundhog Day*'s key lines is uttered by Phil when he is trying to teach Rita, the object of his desire, how to throw cards straight into a hat, some feet away. '*Be* the hat!' he says to her. That statement is pure Zen. One is not to aim at the target 'out there': rather, identify with the target in yourself, so that you and the target become one. In other words, concentrate: for the bullseye will be found there, at your inmost core.

What all the great traditions, including medicine, have in common is a discipline or method. This requires hours of practice. One achieves not only physical perfection but a kind of moral perfection. This requires a degree of humility, a humility that has at its base hard work and good intentions. In this way, one acquires talent that, in the absence of pride, enters the sphere of true virtue. This in turn requires a lack of desire for acknowledgement, or for being praised. It requires that even the subconscious, which carries in it a natural desire for praise, can be governed by a humble goodness, a self-effacement in goodness, which has become second nature. Virtue itself becomes the goal, rather than acting virtuously.

Virtue extends to compassion to everyone one encounters, particularly to those from whom no possible benefit is to be gained. Compassion, like the other virtues, now needs to flow from our very being, irrespective of earthly advantage. In the words of St Bernard, 'Love seeks no cause beyond itself and no fruit; it is its own fruit, its own enjoyment. I love because I love.'

It is important to progress from stage to stage in this quest for virtue as follows:

1. To make oneself virtuous.
2. No longer seeking to be an image of virtue but actually being virtuous.
3. Being virtuous, constantly striving for it, intending it with all our heart, regardless of the consequences of one's actions in the world.
4. To make tomorrow today so that there is no longer any procrastination.

In the Greek orthodox tradition, the spiritual path is described in terms of this metaphor: a man wishes to plant a tree; on his way to the place where he wants to plant it, he stumbles across a treasure and forgets the tree. To explain this metaphor: the transplanting of the tree is our goal, our aim, our intention, our desire; the treasure is the beauty of Human Spirit, which is infinitely greater than anything we could imagine at the start of our quest. Once we understand this, we will begin to glimpse the gleams of this treasure wherever we are, whatever we are doing.

It might not perhaps be out of place to cite here this passage from St Paul's letter to the Philippians:

Brethren, I count not myself to have apprehended: but this one thing I do, forgetting those things which are behind, and reaching forth unto those things which are before, I press toward the mark for the prize of the high calling of God in Christ Jesus.

CHAPTER TWELVE

Introspection – A Return to the Spirit

'Mistah Kurtz—he dead.'
Heart of Darkness by Joseph Conrad

When old age shall this generation waste,
Thou shalt remain, in midst of other woe
Than ours, a friend to man, to whom thou say'st,
'Beauty is truth, truth beauty' – that is all
Ye know on earth, and all ye need to know.
'Ode on a Grecian Urn' by John Keats

Why does anyone wish to study medicine? An individual may wish to study medicine for a variety of reasons, or a combination of reasons. There are different archetypes and combinations of archetypes. There is the 'save the world' archetype – as C.S. Lewis said, 'She is the sort of woman who lives for others – you can tell the others by their hunted expression.' There are those who want to understand how everything works, fascinated by the most incredible workings of the human body. There are those who seek a secure job for life. There are those who cannot think of anything better to do. This list is not exhaustive.

Medicine has a place for everyone. However, a significant proportion of medical students do not finish the course, and a significant proportion will leave the profession after qualification. This is a waste of an enormous amount of resource, both at a personal level and at a national level. The vast majority of leavers do so because there is a failure to meet expectations. Namely, a disillusionment or an increasing maturity that leads to a change of perspective.

What is key is to see medicine as it is. Where I have used anecdotes, this is simply to illustrate points and to present the realities of the subject and profession of medicine.

When Dostoevsky threw out the enigmatic remark 'Beauty will save the world', particularly in the movement of darkness that tends to surround modern living, one could ask the question as Solzhenitsyn did: 'When in bloodthirsty history did beauty ever save anyone or anything? Ennobled, uplifted, yes – but whom has it saved?' He went on to speculate that perhaps Dostoevsky's remark was not a careless phrase, but a prophecy. To lose a sense of beauty is to lose a sense of proportion. To appreciate beauty is first to identify what you may find beautiful, what brings you peace, and then to see things and events in their proper context.

It seems to me that modern existence is spent in front of a screen. A screen, by necessity, is a two-dimensional world. It takes away any perception of depth, both vertically and horizontally.

A two-dimensional view with sight is by definition a loss of heart. Any sense of beauty requires a perception of depth. No wonder then, that life in front of a screen makes one accustomed to a two-dimensional world. We begin to experience not only a loss of visual depth but also a perception of depth. For example, we experience the loss of the ability to understand facial expression. A loss of perception is then an inability to empathise. Already there is concern among educationalists regarding the inability of schoolchildren, whose lives are spent in front of a screen both at home and at school, to express themselves visually by means of facial expression, or to understand facial expression. Most teenagers, having limited insight, would violently disagree. This in itself is sufficient to disconnect one individual from another. The failure is the inability to comprehend that the 'other' is none other than 'I'. Thus, the loss of empathy.

An inability to empathise can be fatal on several levels. In a simple conversation, the incapacity to understand or question the topic can lead to a fruitless discussion. More seriously, an inability to empathise often involves being unable to discern the context of an interaction. A reluctance to engage is also fundamentally selfish, and it can be damaging not to understand the mood or perspective of either an individual or an audience. Being unable to contextualise is the fundamental flaw in the lack of empathy.

At a personal level, the inability to see oneself through the eyes of another is a profound loss, with potentially horrific consequences that can reverberate across generations and society. This is amply exemplified by events that occurred at the Mid Staffordshire NHS Foundation Trust, in which numerous patients who were admitted to hospital with acute conditions faced tremendous abuse at the hands of their carers – including a combination of physicians, clinicians and managers. The public inquiry into this needless suffering at Stafford Hospital concluded that the culture of care that used to exist in the NHS had been replaced by a culture of 'command and control', allowing otherwise caring individuals to become oblivious to the tremendous abuses they were both sanctioning and participating in.

This lack of empathy and the ability to see how others feel or to understand the suffering of another is fundamentally an inability to treat others as one would treat oneself.

Beauty is often said to be in the eye of the beholder. This seems to imply that there are archetypes of beauty or for judging beauty. I think it can be commonly agreed that virgin nature itself would be the archetype, whether it be the sky at night, or the trees in the forests, the mountains, the birds or animals, or indeed a newborn baby. Surely only very few cannot be moved by these, however much of their lives is focused on themselves or their screens. There seems to be an innate trait or knowledge of beauty in each individual that not even a life in front of a screen can take away.

I believe that Dostoevsky was prophetic, particularly in a world where our lives have become increasingly governed by a screen. This is both by necessity and by choice. All purchases can be made online. All information about any detail can be obtained via Google or social media. It is not uncommon to witness people staring into their phones while walking across a street. It has required legislation to stop people looking at a screen while driving!

I also believe that Dostoevsky was prophetic, because beauty is the remedy. It seems to me that a remedy for this increasing reduction of all of life on to a screen is to re-engage with virgin nature, which in my view most fully reveals the archetype of all beauty. It is, at the very least, to discipline oneself and spend as much time as possible away from the screen. A walk outdoors in a park or a garden can change one's entire perspective on life, bringing one back from the abstract and the virtual to the beautiful and the actual – to the beauty of reality. Simply looking at the night sky, gazing at a tree, being inspired by the scent of a flower: such simple things evoke in our spirit the reality of beauty for which we all yearn.

Perhaps best of all, by engaging with someone through the art of conversation, you recall the art of making eye contact and perceiving how others see you, and to perhaps truly see the other. To appreciate depth in facial expression. To empathise. To understand the infinite possibilities in terms of the human condition, human emotion. An ability to share is in itself something beautiful. This is precisely why Dostoevsky declared that 'beauty shall save the world'.

The spiritual beauty inherent in human empathy is brought to light in *Uppada Sutta*, a story from the Pali canon in the Buddhist tradition. The Buddha's leading disciple, Ananda, had engaged in a wonderfully uplifting conversation about the spiritual life with his fellow monks. He then went to the Buddha and, beaming with enthusiasm, declared: 'Lord, this is half of the spiritual life: admirable friendship, admirable companionship, admirable camaraderie.' To which the Buddha replied, 'Say not so, Ananda, say not so. Admirable friendship, admirable companionship, admirable camaraderie is the *whole* of the spiritual life.'

What the Buddha teaches us here is that we cannot place any limits on the graces that come through spiritual companionship, through face-to-face engagement with kindred spirits aiming at the same lofty ideals, desiring nothing more than to give and receive that love which gives wings to the most noble aspirations. No amount of 'virtual' reality, digital communication or social media can replace the spiritual nourishment provided by real, interpersonal engagement (*satsang*, in the Hindu and Buddhist traditions; *suhba* in the Muslim tradition).

* * *

A darkness has crept into the art, science and practice of medicine. Medicine, which has always been a means of delivering care, has been destroyed, becoming an end in itself. Doctors have become obsessed with delivery and have forgotten care. This is precisely the conclusion reached by the Francis Report into the abuse that occurred at Stafford Hospital, and which is now known to have also occurred at many other centres. How is it possible for elderly patients to lie in corridors for hours on end in their own excrement? This is the same horror that was described by Kurtz in Joseph Conrad's *Heart of Darkness*, although at least in that story Kurtz ultimately recognises the horror of his position and determines to remove everything, including himself, that was part of the process that led to it. This darkness is endemic and requires not radical surgery, but a return to the spirit of care.

An underlying cause of this malaise is an obsession with delivery, with commissioning, with process, with algorithms, and a forgetfulness of (or at least an inadvertence to) the subject matter of all of this. The human being. The human state. The answer to the nature of the malaise that lies within the heart of the medical system.

The remedy is to realise that the nature of the malaise that lies within the heart of the medical system has engendered this horror. The horror starts with an inappropriate humanitarianism that puts form before substance. The laudable aim of setting up the National Health Service to deliver care to everyone, irrespective of means, free at the point of delivery, has degenerated to the culture of command and control.

The remedy also lies within the heart and the spirit. The heart of our society, and in the heart of every individual. The archetype of all beauty is glimpsed in virgin nature. The quintessence of virgin nature is the human being, both form and substance. The most beautiful of all within the quintessence of virgin nature is the substance or the spirit of the being. Therein lies the answer: beauty shall save the world.

• • •

It was a warm autumn night in early October. A curious glow emanated from the street lamps on Broad Street in Oxford, reflecting on the college walls and bathing the street in a dull yellow light.

A student crossed over to gain the night entrance to his college. The gloom reflected his disheartened mood. His day had started with the unusual experience of having a tutorial, one to one. He found this rather frightening, as it had previously been possible to hide in the anonymity of a class and avoid eye contact with his teachers. He had been asked to prepare an essay for his tutorial and had undertaken, in the usual fashion, an eighteen-page document rehashing and citing all of the latest sources, making up an elaborate answer to what seemed an elaborate question. He was shocked to the core at being asked what he *thought* after having regurgitated what he had *read*, and found himself stumbling, unable to provide an original answer. Consequently, he had received a B from his tutor, who told him he was perfectly aware of what had already been written on the subject. All his tutor wanted was two pages about what the student thought. This had unnerved him.

The final straw had been his attendance at the Improvisation Society of the university. He had bought a reed flute. He had never played one but loved the instrument and its mournful sound. He understood the lament of the reed flute, a symbol of the soul's sorrow at being parted from its origin. He had in his mind these lines, as a paraphrase of the lines of the opening of the *Mathnawi* of the thirteenth-century Persian poet and Sufi mystic, Rumi:

If you wish to know how lovers bleed,
Listen my friend, listen, to the reed.
It speaks of separation.

Everyone sundered far from his origin longs to recapture the time when he was united with it. This is what the student felt in his bones, and he was wondering how and when he would find the path that would lead him back to his home. But his nostalgic yearning was not to be satisfied by what he heard at the Improvisation Society. He experienced the most ghastly noise, enough to destroy any ear sensitive to music.

Having crossed Broad Street, the student experienced an apparition. A lanky and bespectacled youth whom he recognised as a fellow member of his college, dressed in black tie, a velvet-collared long coat and a top hat. What was remarkable was that he was in the process of vigorously fencing the lamp post that stood near the entrance with a silver-tipped cane. The dull yellow glow bathed his white tie and starched dicky in a ghostly luminescence.

The student, flute in hand, dressed in his anorak, was filled with a sense of wonder. 'What are you doing?' he asked.

'Can you not see that I am fencing this lamp post?' the other responded, as if this were the most natural activity in the world.

I engaged with my fellow student. He in his tails, and me in my anorak. Each of us from entirely different backgrounds and perspectives, but united in our love of fencing. The student, whose name was Simon, informed me that he had fenced for his school, as had I. We decided to go and drink vast amounts of coffee in his room and he sobered up considerably. We then had a long conversation, lasting the rest of the night and into the early hours of the morning, again fortified by coffee, on the very subject of beauty and art.

Simon and I became firm friends and he was the best man at my wedding. Our views were disparate, both politically and philosophically, although we were great allies in union politics at Oxford. We have since become closer over the years but he remains a committed agnostic and I still don't think we see eye to eye from a philosophical perspective.

Thus began my pursuit of beauty. I became aware, in a way that cannot be fully articulated, that a sense of alienation and bewilderment is actually the beginning of the spiritual quest. It tells the soul that the search for meaning, for ultimate truth, is in fact a search for the absolute source of beauty. I felt that, however baffling be this world into which I was entering, there would always be a further stage of bewilderment, that stage evoked by Rumi in the lament of the reed, uprooted, separated, longing for return to its home. I also felt that the greater the bewilderment, the greater the yearning for beauty; and the greater the thirst for beauty, the greater the anticipation, the presentiment, the foretaste: the essence of beauty is already, mysteriously, 'tasted' in the very thirst of our bewildered longing.

According to Rumi, the soul that yearns for God, calling upon Him day and night, eventually hears this response: 'That need, that pain, that burning of yours is Our message to you.'

* * *

Justice, which is none other than the expression of truth on all levels, penetrates the whole world, as there is bound to be for every action a concordant reaction. 'There is no right superior to that of the Truth', according to the sages of Benares, to which we must add the Platonic maxim: 'Beauty is the splendour of the Truth.' When beauty and truth come together, justice will be born: a resonance that reverberates through every echelon of society.

Britain has traditionally been characterised by its system of justice, the rule of law. A robust system that renders corruption, with its very beginning, falsehood, difficult to thrive. In the same way, Keats tells us that beauty penetrates the world, and, as it does so, elicits a response in the same way that truth does. He explains that in a society where truth reverberates, this is none other than beauty, and beauty is characterised by a purity that is akin to truth, for they are, at root, indistinguishable. For man and the human condition, beauty is at one with the ultimate truth and with infinite goodness. The reality to which truth bears witness is beauty and goodness infinite.

Every stakeholder, when taking ownership of an interactional process, needs to have a period of introspection. Every patient and every doctor needs to introspect to reach their goal: a doctor to deliver the best care possible; the patient to get an outcome that manages their expectation. This implies both an individual mission and a common ownership from the initial consultation to the final discharge, whatever the outcome, working either as a collective or as an individual.

So how can this be achieved? I go first to a collective means of taking ownership. The best example that has been tried and tested throughout the ages is the 'Twelve Steps' of curing addiction. Unfortunately, many clinicians don't like it because it excludes them; equally, many clinicians don't like it because it brings into the mix God or some godlike figure. So what are the Twelve Steps? Let us start with the Twelve Steps of Narcotics Anonymous. We are, after all, in the middle of an opioid epidemic, which has killed more Americans in recent times than any war – as previously mentioned, the majority from prescription drugs as opposed to illicit drugs.

My own experience of the value of the Twelve Steps came to me in a curious way. I shared a room at Oxford with a close friend, in a house in Jericho, together with another friend; when we moved to London, me as a junior doctor, he as a banker, we shared his flat in south London, together with his most wonderful then girlfriend (to whom I remain close today). Unbeknown to both of us, he was an opiate addict. The first we knew of it was when his father informed us that he had disclosed his son's addiction to the bank, and that they were going to pay for his rehabilitation. Part of this was to completely sever all his relationships, including with his girlfriend (who I don't think ever recovered), and although he remains someone I see from time to time, we do not share the friendship we once had. However, I think NA and the Twelve Steps saved his life.

The Twelve Steps of Narcotics Anonymous are:

1. We admitted that we were powerless over our addiction, that our lives had become unmanageable.
2. We came to believe that a power greater than ourselves could restore us to sanity.
3. We made a decision to turn our will and our lives over to the care of a power greater than ourselves.
4. We made a searching and fearless moral inventory of ourselves.
5. We admitted to a power greater than ourselves, to ourselves and to another human being the exact nature of our wrongs.
6. We were entirely ready to have a power greater than ourselves remove all these defects of character.
7. We humbly ask a power greater than ourselves to remove our shortcomings.
8. We made a list of all persons we had harmed, and became willing to make amends to them all.
9. We made direct amends to such people wherever possible, except when to do so would injure them or others.
10. We continued to take personal inventory, and when we were wrong, promptly admitted it.
11. We sought through prayer and meditation to improve our conscious contact with a power greater than ourselves as we

understood it, praying only for knowledge of that which for us will give us the power to carry that out.
12. Having had a spiritual awakening as a result of these steps, we tried to carry this message to addicts, and to practise these principles in all our affairs.

These steps can be taken by all of us, whatever our 'addiction' may be, whatever be the form taken by our particular kind of idolatry: money, power, lust, vanity. Or whatever form be taken by our particular kind of obsession or mental or emotional imbalance. The greatest and most obvious imbalance we see around us is in the relationship between the self and the 'other'.

There needs to be reintegration of the self with the other – beginning with that transcendent other. At an interpersonal level, between the self and one's family, and colleagues and friends; and at an ecological level, between one's inner world and virgin nature.

The macrocosm is reflected in the microcosm and vice versa. If we can put right what is wrong with our little world, the effect upon the outer world is incalculable.

* * *

It is often said that doctors tend to marry other doctors or other healthcare professionals, as it is only they who can understand the context in which healthcare professionals work. It is often said that the reward for hard work within the healthcare system is more hard work. This is never more so than in the medicine, where the demonstration that one can work hard is simply rewarded by more stringent targets.

It is sad to see so many colleagues whose personal lives have deteriorated with their partners or their children because they have either made a value judgement not to spend the time or make the effort or indeed have, for the purposes of financial need or choice, been precluded from doing so. Every being needs buttons pressed to function integrally. A child needs the buttons of responsible parenthood. Often, they also need the buttons of responsible grandparenthood. These are important in terms of establishing behaviour, role models and much more, all of which are the subject of many other books and not the purpose of this book. Ultimately, charity begins at home and starts with charity to one's true self. Once one has had the inclination to spend time alone with oneself, it becomes easier to integrate oneself with others. Once home life is harmonious, it becomes easier to create harmony in one's relationships with colleagues and patients. What is required is not a compartmentalised life, but one that is integral and consistent. One can only have such an integral life when one is true to oneself. As Polonius said in his last piece of advice to his son Laertes in Shakespeare's *Hamlet*: 'This above all: to thine own self be true. And it must follow, as the night the day, thou canst not then be false to any man.' But then, how do we find our true self?

The Buddha tells us, most enigmatically, that there is no true self: *anatta*, no-self, is at the heart of his enlightenment. We can understand this to mean that we must not identify ourselves with anything that is transient, any self-conception that fixates on a passing aspect of our consciousness; for anything that passes away cannot be true: the only reality is that which is eternal, and this eternal reality of our 'self' can only be seen through the state of enlightenment. Short of this, it can be intuited by the heart, to the extent that the seeker is sincerely following the Noble Eightfold Path taught by the Buddha. In other words, the eye of the heart opens up in the very measure that we are putting 'right' everything about our lives:

1. Right understanding
2. Right thinking
3. Right speaking
4. Right acting
5. Right livelihood
6. Right effort
7. Right mindfulness
8. Right concentration

When all these dimensions of our life are in their right place, then there will be justice, harmony, beauty and truth. The spiritual state of consciousness attained in the Buddha's enlightenment is one in which there is no room for any consciousness of anything apart from the essence of consciousness itself.

The Buddha was so perplexed by the cycle of birth, old age, disease and death that he could no longer contain himself in his palace as the young Prince Siddhartha with his family, and had to leave to find an answer to this conundrum. He retreated to virgin nature as he understood that the answer to any conundrum or remedy to any ailment lay therein, and in the virgin nature of human consciousness. It is said that he mastered the language of the birds. He understood the words of the wind. Yet he found no answers. He wandered the forests alone, deep in meditation, studying every aspect of nature. Eventually, he went to a river and saw a reflection of himself. He understood at that point that the answers he sought were to be found in the universe that lay within him. He understood that within every atom was a mystery opening out to the Absolute and the Infinite. He understood that truth consisted of not only a 'yes' or a 'no', but also of infinite possibilities. He understood that he was a reflection of the universe; that nirvana was none other than the consciousness within him. These truths became enshrined in his heart by his enlightenment under the fig tree, when his consciousness and the reality of nirvana were one.

The notion of togetherness within oneness is expressed, in an interesting way, by contemporary Rastafarians. To them, 'I' means 'me'. 'I and I' means 'we', in that the other is none other than 'I'. 'I and I and I' is the universal consciousness that pervades us all. This is what is achieved by introspection or meditation, in understanding not only one's own consciousness but that all consciousness, and therefore all beings, are connected. This is precisely the same as the saying of Christ, 'Love thy neighbour as thyself'.

All four of the Buddha's 'noble truths' are concerned with suffering: its reality, its cause, its termination and the path to its termination. We are all suffering in one way or another, we are all deficient in some respect: only the holy ones are fully healthy, the rest of us are suffering from some form of disease, even if it be only in the sense of dis-ease – in other words, an absence of ease, comfort, contentment and inner peace.

To remedy any disease or dis-ease, it is important to find the cause. Nowhere more so than in the management of physical pain.

Pain is often somatised. In other words, there could be either an emotional or a physical cause of pain. Often it is both. Just as outward pain can be the result of a particular psychological state, so a particular psychological state can be the cause of the neutralisation of physical pain. We see many instances of this during war, for example. Many of us have read about the famous exchange during the Battle of Waterloo where the Duke of Wellington was seated next to his second in command, Lord Paget. Both were on horseback, watching the battle unfold in front of them, when a shell landed nearby.

Lord Paget glanced down and said, 'By God, sir, I've lost a leg!'

To which Lord Wellington replied, 'By God, sir, so you have!'

Pain not only has a generator but can also be understood in terms of the subjective perception of pain. When one is in a good mood or on an adrenaline high, one might hardly feel pain. When one is depressed or in a bad mood, one may feel the same pain – objectively, the same generator – but experience it subjectively in a much more acute or severe form.

Pain, if it remains present for a long time, becomes a memory, a 'phantom'. This happens at the level of the spinal cord (where there are now treatments of spinal cord stimulation to try to eradicate this memory), or even at the level of the brain (where there are now brain stimulators to do the same). Either way, this 'centralisation' of pain means that the pain has ceased to be at the level of where it is being generated and has moved into the nervous system. At this stage, even removing the cause of the pain will no longer remove the perception of it, which has become very much part of the brain or nervous system. The longer something generates pain, the more likely that it becomes 'phantom'.

Phantom pain or central pain cannot be solved by means of opiates. And even though they do appear to work, they only give temporary relief, never a permanent cure. After a while you get used to the level of opiates, which then must keep on being increased. This can cause depression, anxiety and hallucinations, and may lead someone to take their own life. We have to break the vicious cycle somewhere. Removing the pain generator, if it is done quickly, would be one way of doing it, but once pain is established, this becomes less of an option. It would need another approach, perhaps that of Narcotics Anonymous, where one effectively learns to live with one's perception of pain. This requires a belief, or at least a belief system.

It was once said that if God didn't exist then it would be necessary to invent Him/Her. After being asked whether he believed in God, one rather thoughtful agnostic replied: 'No, but I have a God-shaped hole in my heart.' In its own way, this proves a point: the human heart, the essence of our consciousness, is so constructed that it cannot function properly – healthily, let us say – without a belief in something transcendent, something absolute, the source of being: whatever be the name one gives it. Here, let us recall the following words from the first chapter of the *Tao Te Ching*: 'A name that can be named is not The Name. Tao is both Named and Nameless. As Nameless, it is the origin of all things; as Named it is the mother of all things.'

There needs to be some form of belief or faith at the core of one's consciousness. When the object of belief is not in something greater than oneself, then, by default, one will only have to believe in oneself: the ego becomes absolutised, and, even if subconsciously, 'worshipped' as a kind of idol. In the Hindu tradition, a strong distinction is drawn between the ordinary self (*jivatman*) and the Supreme Self (*paramatman*). We can understand this Self as a universal level of consciousness, which does not belong to my little ego, rather in the way that a wave belongs to the ocean, not the ocean to the wave. And my little wave of consciousness, when it discovers the vastness of the ocean to which it belongs, realises that its strength is nothing compared to the tidal waves of power that can be generated by the ocean. The wave is part of this vast ocean, it is never separate from it, but the question is, how to tap into its immense power? Without the ocean, the power of my tiny wave is negligible, but with the power of the ocean, no obstacle is insurmountable.

One of the reasons why the Twelve Steps emphasise so much the need for belief in something that infinitely transcends the ego is that addicts normally have a gut feeling that, on their own, they are helpless. They know, viscerally, that they need something super-human. Mahayana Buddhists call this something 'Other-Power' (*tariki*), the power of the absolutely Other, as opposed to the power of the self (*jiriki*).

There needs to be an introspection, a thinking, a meditation, which the Twelve Step programme initiates through collective meditation. Any form of communal or group activity is a start, but it is intended to initiate, for each individual, a process of some form of systematic introspection, some form of meditation, some deeper mode of what religious people call 'prayer'. There are many belief systems that incorporate this introspection into their practice. All of them would emphasise the primacy of this introspection over any external form of worship. Or, at least, they would concur in saying that the externals of worship require sincerity, which in turn requires inner purification, hence introspection and total honesty about oneself – one's faults and weaknesses. The addict will gradually come to the realisation: as I begin to unravel the knots of my character, I begin to uncover the hidden roots of my addiction. The greater the insight into myself, the more focused will be my effort to uproot those faults of my character that led to my alienation from my true self, and from there to my vulnerability: my fall into the pit of addiction. And getting out of this pit? This is where faith is crucial. The addict will understand: the drug was a demon pretending to be my saviour; but now I am liberated from that false god, not through my own limited resources, but through the infinite power that becomes available to me, in proportion to my faith in the source of all power, being and – let us add – beauty.

Let us then look at the Twelve Steps again.

1. They admit that they have a problem. This means admitting that they, on their own, have become unable to manage it. When an addict gets up at a meeting, the first thing he says is his name, to acknowledge himself, followed by the statement, 'I am an addict'. He acknowledges both his state as an individual and an articulation of his problem. To understand the disease is to begin to understand the remedy.
2. They put faith in the existence of a higher power. This is a process that could restore them to good health. The Buddha said: 'Good health is the greatest gift.'
3. They resolve to put themselves in the hands of a higher power. Their cure and thus their lives are handed over to either a collective or a process.
4. They make an inventory of themselves. This means carrying out a systematic study of their own symptoms and of their expectations.
5. They admit the nature of their 'wrongs'. This means admitting to the collective the exact nature of their problems and their expectations.
6. They are willing to have a higher power remove their 'defects'. This means handing over their 'cure' as far as possible to the other, understanding what the other can do for them, and any limitations.
7. They ask a higher power to remove their shortcomings. They realise that this whole process requires a degree of humility and understanding of their shortcomings.
8. They consider any harm they have caused to other people. It is important to understand the context of illness and who else might be involved in the care of the individual, and how they might be affected. There needs to be a comprehensive vision of their illness in the context of their lives.
9. They make amends for any harm they have caused. An individual's cure will require support from all those who are either

dependent on the individual, or who care for the individual. This may be something as simple as arranging for the care of a pet, or childcare for a single parent. There needs to be an acknowledgement of what everyone has done in this process, and has given to this process. This may include family members but also includes the carers – for example, the doctors, and the whole team involved in the management of a disease.

10. They maintain their moral inventory. This involves a comprehensive personal inventory requiring candour on the part of the individual, whether he be the doctor or the patient.
11. They maintain contact with a higher power. This requires a constant process of introspection, managing at each stage expectation and matching it with outcome.
12. They practise these principles in all their affairs and carry their message to other addicts. Having mastered the process of introspection, the final step is to communicate this through patient organisations, and there are many such organisations. It is important that these patient organisations are an integral part of any provider. In this way, patients can communicate their experiences to each other, but also these organisations (a collective) can communicate with the provider, which can only lead to a better care pathway.

There has to be a return to a model of care and the focus should not be 'targets' but that of the care pathway. This will inevitably emphasise the pre-eminence of care over that of control. It will also ensure that whenever change is effected, the primary aim is to give better care. Better care is delivered by better managing expectations and by improving outcomes.

• • •

It is imperative, in all circumstances of life, to orient oneself to transcendent beauty. This is simply another way of doing what Jesus tells us to do in the first great commandment: to love God with all our heart, all our soul, all our mind and all our strength. This is why mystics of all the world's great spiritual traditions are unanimous in affirming that all the beauties that surround us – the beauty of nature, the beauty of sacred art and architecture, the beauty of the souls around us, the beauty of the human face, in all its infinite variety – all of these forms and expressions of beauty are to be found within our heart, understood as the core, the source, the essence of our human consciousness. It is in our own hearts that we can reconnect with the source of beauty.

Turning within, through mindfulness, introspection, meditation, invocation – prayer in all its forms – is our most fundamental way of reconnecting with the source of beauty within ourselves. When we begin to sense this inner beauty, two rather marvellous things are set in motion within us: firstly, we begin to see more clearly everything in our soul – our character, our conduct, our attitudes, our intentions – that is not in harmony with this beauty. In the light of beauty, we see more clearly our own ugliness. But, more importantly, we are empowered to do something about it, motivated not just by some external rule of conduct, but by an inner imperative: an overpowering need to make ourselves conform in all respects with the beauty of the Real. A need born out of the depths of the love we have for that beauty.

Secondly, in proportion to our sense of the beauty within us, we begin to see, with the eye of the heart, traces of that beauty outside us, all around us. We begin to see the beauties of virgin nature: 'Wherever ye turn, there is the Face of God', as the Qur'an tells us. Then, with our heightened sensitivity to the beauty of nature –

whether it be a tree, a flower, a bird or any animal – one is much more likely to want to save it, to preserve it, and to respect it, doing so out of a sense of belonging to the self-same beauty that these phenomena of nature manifest. Our solidarity with Mother Nature will be deepened the more profoundly we feel our oneness with Her in the beauty of Reality.

This process of discovery, this unfolding of saving beauty, can start simply by resolutely turning off one's computer, switching off one's mobile phone, and taking a long walk in the park; by looking at the star-filled sky at night; or by gazing at the flight of a flock of birds.

The wonderful and complex workings of nature are the most poignant reminder of one's place in it. Mother Nature makes us aware of our limitations and our tininess within this immensity, but She also shows us that the source of all Her power and beauty is to be found within our own hearts. If we can reconnect with that beauty within, we will open ourselves up to that miraculous grace of being healed, in the spiritual sense of the word. We open ourselves up to finding that 'pearl of great price', that 'peace that surpasses all understanding', of which Jesus spoke. We open ourselves up to that priceless gift: imperturbable serenity.

St Seraphim of Sarov famously told one of his disciples: 'Find inner peace, and thousands around you will find their salvation.' And one can only find this inner peace through being liberated from the prison of one's own egotism. Where there is egotism, selfishness, greed, materialism, vanity, pride, ambition and ostentation, there will always be agitation, dispersion, anxiety, insatiability and discontent, however hard one tries to repress these symptoms of dis-ease through distractions, obsessions and driving ambitions.

• • •

One deeper meaning of the saying 'Charity begins at home' is that we can only begin to do good to others if we have ourselves become good. And we can only be good if we are liberated from the pride of thinking that we are good, and realising the truth of Jesus's words: 'Why callest thou me good? There is none good but one, that is, God.' God's goodness will flow through us, only insofar as we eliminate our egotism.

If we truly begin to change ourselves in our quest not just to see beauty, but to conform to beauty, an immense power may well be unleashed: a power that has nothing to do with us, and everything to do with beauty. The more deeply we understand this, the more earnestly we will strive for self-effacement and humility, generosity and compassion, patience and discipline, sincerity and justice – seeing these virtues as so many beauties of soul. Each of us can become an artist in this sense: making a work of art out of our own souls. Doing this through truth, virtue and meditation is the greatest thing we can do both for ourselves and for the world.

If beauty is to save the world, we have to see to it that beauty first saves us. Beauty can then, through analogical magic, save those around us. This relationship between our own resolve to change ourselves and the capacity of others around us to change themselves for the better is hugely important. By taking control of our own lives, a positive influence comes through us (rather than from us), an influence that can transform the lives of others around us, including the life pulsatingly present in virgin nature. Engaging with the beauty outside us has to start by bringing to light the beauty within.

* * *

So, should my children read medicine? The answer is an unqualified, unreserved and totally enthusiastic: 'Yes'. Despite the darkness that I have described descending upon the profession of modern medicine, if my children have a sincere desire to alleviate the suffering of others, to care for them with compassion, and to find fulfilment in the ancient and honourable art of healing, how could I possibly try to dissuade them?

Of course, I would insist they enter the profession with their eyes open to the prevailing abuses and to the obstacles in their way. They will need a clear mind and a strong will to ensure that their noble intentions will be realised. They must know that they will be confronting a system of medicinal care that is increasingly at odds with its own reason for being. But, when all is said and done, the medical system is managed and run by individuals, by human beings, who cannot but be sensitive to those qualities – care, compassion, love, empathy – that enter into the very definition of our humanity. Even if the policies, systems and institutions under which they work are drifting into the very opposite of those qualities – command and control – we cannot place any limits on the impact that just one doctor can make, a single doctor in whom the science of medicine is skilfully blended with the art of healing.

There is also the prospect that the efforts of individuals will be complemented and reinforced by new collective initiatives. There appears to be something of a seismic shift among venture capitalists, those prepared to put money into new ventures to support what are known as 'high impact' ventures – ventures that would have a high impact at a social level. These seem to be a great deal more valued these days than ventures that are capable of deriving 'derivatives' of a financial system that seems to be in deep trouble. It is therefore possible in this day and age to be an 'entrepreneur' in a social sense, by being paid to deliver care.

I cannot help thinking at this point of my mother, who always wished me to be a doctor, but was scandalised when she heard that

I was actually being paid to deliver care! Whenever I returned to Sri Lanka on vacation after I had qualified as a doctor, large numbers of people would be standing outside my house, sometimes for hours, in order to receive my opinion and treatment free of charge. My mother would insist that every single one of them should not only be seen, diagnosed and treated, but also fed, watered and conversed with. You can imagine the amount of time this took, and on occasion much of my vacation was spent doing this. I didn't have the heart to refuse her, and every time I would raise my voice in complaint, she would look at me in a censorial way and warn me about the curse of money. This struck me somewhat as being at odds with the work of my father, who was an outright businessman and who traded profitably. She seemed to have no objection to him earning as much as he could with respect to his trade. She simply felt that since I had been born to a degree of wealth, my skills should be dispensed for free, and that my sole reward should be the satisfaction of helping to cure the sick and help the needy. As well as reminding me of the reason I wanted to be a doctor, my mother was teaching me the principle of *noblesse oblige*!

I am pleased to say that modern venture capital and entrepreneurship sees things differently. In fact, the ability to provide high-impact care that makes a difference to people's lives is much valued, and people are beginning to invest in the ability to do this. I therefore think that it is possible to deliver care, as care should be delivered, *and* be properly paid. Nonetheless, the spirit underlying my mother's attitude taught me something infinitely more precious than any amount of money. She taught me that the giving of care, with compassion and empathy, seeking no material reward for myself, actually helps me to enter into the fullness of my own humanity. I discovered that, by helping others to overcome sickness and be restored to health, and by enabling them to fulfil their human potential, I was doing something much more important than just earning a wage. I was participating in the most uplifting and satisfying work of all: engaging with my fellow human beings in an exploration of the limitless potential of the human condition when it is restored to health and wholeness.

* * *

I started this chapter with an anecdote about a lamp post and it is appropriate to finish now with another. This comes from the corpus of legends surrounding Mulla Nasruddin, a kind of 'holy fool' whose antics masked profound wisdom. One night, he is seen by a neighbour searching for something under lamplight in the street. He asks Mulla what he is looking for.

'My key,' Mulla says.

The neighbour duly gets down on his hands and knees and starts looking. After some time, he says, 'Mulla, are you sure you dropped your key here?'

'Oh no,' comes the reply, 'I lost my key at home.'

The puzzled neighbour then asks Mulla why he is looking under this lamp.

'Because it's dark at home, there is more light here,' Mulla replies.

This story can be interpreted in a number of ways. This is how I understand it. The key opens the door to beauty. That is what we are all looking for. But we are all looking for it in the outer world ('the street') rather than in our own heart ('home'). Why? Because when we look into our hearts we see that it is 'dark' in comparison with the light that helps us to see things in the world. But once we have quietened down the noisiness of our mind, arrived at a little silence and stillness within, excluding the images coming in from the outside world, we may begin to penetrate the darkness that enshrouds the mystery of our heart. We may begin to sense, or even to glimpse, the infinite beauty that is opened up by the key of the heart. We may come to understand, either gradually or at once, that all the beauties in the world, without exception, are to be found, in their fullness, in those unfathomable depths unlocked within us. We may come to see something of the beauty of 'Layla': her name, 'the night', being the most apt symbol used by the Sufis to hint at that ultimate mystery, the hidden Essence of the Real. Then we may be able to sing, with the Lady Wisdom, symbolised by the Shulamite maiden in Solomon's *Song of Songs*, 'I am black, but beautiful'.

And an entire world may be saved.

* * *

It is my most fervent hope that this book will encourage many young people who are entering the medical profession, helping them to nurture the culture of compassionate care that used to exist in the NHS, which is at the heart of the healing profession, and which goes to the root of what makes us human.

Bibliography

I acknowledge the invaluable contribution of Dr Reza Shah-Kazemi in reading my script and in providing me with appropriate quotes from Schuon, Lings and other sacred texts, and for his analysis of the film *Groundhog Day*.

Ancient Beliefs & Modern Superstitions, Martin Lings (Mandala Books, 1991)

The Big Society, Jesse Norman (University of Buckingham Press, November 2010)

'Epidemic of Deaths from Fentanyl Overdose', *British Medical Journal*, October 2017

The Eye of the Heart, Frithjof Schuon (Bloomington: World Wisdom, 1997)

The Francis Report (Report of the Mid-Staffordshire NHS Foundation Trust public inquiry), Robert Francis QC, February 2013

Getting It Right First Time (GIRFT), Professor Tim Briggs, 2012

Heart of Darkness, Joseph Conrad (first published in *Blackwood's* magazine, 1899)

'The Hollow Men', T.S. Eliot, in *Poems 1909–1925* (Harcourt, Brace & Co, 1925)

The House of God, Samuel Shem (Black Swan, 1978)

Mathnawi Of Jalal Al-Din Rumi, Arberry, A.J. (trans.) (London, John Murray, 1961)

'Ode on a Grecian Urn', John Keats, in *Poetry* (1820)

A Return to the Spirit, Martin Lings (Louisville, US: Fons Vitae, 2005)

Tao Te Ching, Star, Jonathan (trans.) (New York: Tarcher, Cornerstone/Penguin, 2001)

WHO International Classification of Disease (ICD), 1967

Index

accountability 47, 49, 98, 105, 110
Adam's Peak 88–9
addiction 67, 124–6, 131–4
Alcoholics Anonymous 67
algorithms xi, 43, 66, 70, 82, 84–5, 86, 87, 120
Ali, Imam 22
Ananda 119
appraisals 39–40
approach surgeons 31, 41

Bandaranaike, S.W.R.D. 37
Battle of Waterloo 129–30
beauty 21–3, 51–2, 57, 89, 100, 115, 116, 118–19, 120, 123–4, 135–6, 137
bedside manner 19–20
Benares, sages of 123
Bentley, Professor George 7, 8, 29–30, 31–2
Bernard, St 113
Black Elk 100–1
blame culture 42–3
body language 83, 85
Briggs, Professor Tim 46, 47
Buddha 119, 127–9, 132
Buddhism 88, 89, 113, 119, 132
budgets 50, 96–7, 104–5, 106, 107–8

care xi, 99–100, 102–10, 117, 134, 138, 139
Care Quality Commission 56
Centers for Disease Control and Prevention (CDC) 54–5

Chapman, Jens 33
chief executives 39, 44, 47
China 75–6
Christianity 18, 88–9
clinicians 39, 46, 47–8, 49, 71, 73, 83, 92, 98, 104, 107, 124
Collins, Jane 97
command and control 37–8, 43, 46, 90–110, 117, 120, 138
commissioning groups 45–6
communication 64–5, 67–70, 83–5, 134
compassion xi, xii, 99–100, 113, 138, 139
compliance 91, 92, 93–4, 95–6, 98
Conrad, Joseph 90, 102, 115, 120
consultants 30, 32, 39, 41–2, 91, 92, 104
consultations 35, 65–6, 73, 83, 85, 97, 124
conversation 34–6, 82, 83, 86–7, 119
COVID-19 (coronavirus SARS-CoV-2) xiii, 75–9

delivery, obsession with 120
Department of Health 97
development 103
divisions 93–4
doctors, 'difficult' 44, 95
Dostoevsky, Fyodor 116, 118, 119
drugs misuse 54–6, 124–6
Duthie, Robert 6–8

Edgar, Michael 57
Eliot, T.S. 37, 64, 82
emotions: emotional states 66–7, 70
  medicalisation of 84, 85–6
empathy 16, 19, 25, 36, 82, 117–18, 119, 138, 139
European Working Time Directive 31
examinations 26–7, 31–2
expectations 45, 49–50, 71, 72–3, 105, 108, 109, 124, 134

facial expressions 20, 116–17, 119
fear, culture of 43, 91, 94
fellowships 20, 25, 32
Fleming, Alexander 3
Francis Report 43, 46, 120
Freud, Sigmund 19

general practices 38–9
GMC, 'Good Medical Practice' 91–2
God 22, 51, 114, 123, 124, 131, 135, 137
Google 118
GPs 38–9, 64–6, 71, 85
Great Ormond Street 94–7
Groundhog Day 110, 111–13

hakim 100
Hanson, Ted 33
Harborview Medical Center 32–3
Harley Street 60
Helali, Badreddin 111, 112
Hinduism 88, 89, 119, 131
hospitals 38–9, 40, 41, 44–7, 68, 92, 96–7
Human Spirit 114
Hunter, Sister 62

ICD (International Classification of Disease) 70, 84
intuition 16, 17, 22–3, 26, 43
Islam 88–9, 100, 119

Jesus 52, 114, 129, 135, 136, 137
John Lewis 102–3
junior doctors 31, 78, 93, 97
justice 123–4

Keats, John 115, 123–4
Kelly, Rachel xii–xiii
Kirwan, Ernie 57, 59–60, 61

Lewis, C.S. 115
Lings, Dr Martin 52–3
litigation 42–3, 45, 48–50, 72

Mahayana Buddhists 132
managers 38, 39, 43–4, 46, 47–8, 49, 93–6, 98–9
Mann, Horace 3
Marks, Charlie 28, 29
Marx, Karl 65
MDT (Multi-Disciplinary Team) 40–1, 50, 82–3, 87, 92
medical training 15–36, 43, 105, 108–9, 115–16
medicine men 100
Mid Staffordshire NHS Foundation Trust 43, 117
Middlesex Hospital 40, 57–8, 94
Moorfields Hospital 59
Morriss-Kay, Gillian 17–18
Mother Nature 136
Muhammad, Prophet 22, 51
Murray, Bill 111, 112–13

Narcotics Anonymous 67, 124–6, 130, 131–4
Nasruddin, Mulla 140–1
National Health Service (NHS) 38–47, 62, 72, 91–2, 98–100, 103, 104, 106–7, 120
National Hospital for Neurology and Neurosurgery 26–8
National Institute of Clinical Excellence 106
Native Americans 100
Noble, Denis 17, 18
Norman, Jesse 102

Northwick Park Hospital 24–5
Nuffield Orthopaedic Centre 6

obesity 106
Oglala Sioux 100–1
opioid misuse 54–6, 124–6
outcomes 28, 45–6, 49–50, 73, 105, 107–8, 109, 124, 134
ownership, taking 41, 86–7, 103, 104, 105, 107, 108, 124
Oxford University 4–8, 13–14, 15–16, 17–18, 19

Paget, Lord 129–30
pain 129–30
Pasteur, Louis 3
patience 62–3
Paul, St 114
phantom pain 130
Phizackerley, Paddy 17, 18
progress 103

quality of care 47–8, 56, 72, 99
Qur'an 135

Ransford, Andrew 57, 60
Rastafarians 129
RCA (Root Cause Analysis) 42–3, 92
relationships, healthcare professionals' 33, 126–7
religion 52–3, 65, 87–9
research 33–4
revision surgery 48
Royal College of Surgeons 20, 32, 57
Royal National Orthopaedic Hospital 29–30, 31–2, 48, 57
Rumi 121, 123

St Mary's Hospital 25
St Thomas' Hospital 28–9
Schuon, Frithjof 100–1
Seraphim of Sarov, St 136
serendipity 2–12
Shah-Kazemi, Reza xii

Shakespeare, William 2, 21, 82, 127
shamanistic societies 100
Shem, Samuel 24, 25
SHO (senior house officer) 30, 32, 41
Simon 121–3
social care, adult 56–7
social media 68, 83–4, 86–7, 107, 118
Solomon 141
Solzhenitsyn, Aleksandr 116
spiritual path 114
Sri Lanka 88–9, 139
Stafford Hospital 46, 117, 120
Stalin, Joseph 98, 99
Sufis 112, 121, 141
surgeons 20, 41, 51, 56
Sutherland, Bryony xiii
Swedish Hospital 32–3
Sweetnam, Sir Rodney 57–8
Symon, Professor Lindsay 26–8

Tao Te Ching 131
targets 39, 46, 56, 72, 93, 99, 126, 134
technology 68–9, 116–17, 118
Thatcher, Margaret 62
Trotsky, Leon 99
Trump, Donald 54, 75
'Twelve Steps' of curing addiction 124–6, 131–4

University College Hospital 57, 62
Uppada Sutta 119

vaccines 76
Vishnu 89
vivisection 34

Walpole, Horace 3
Walter Mercer Gold Medal 32
Wellington, Duke of 129–30
WHO, Surgical Safety Checklist 92, 93, 105–6